C000101068

This book has been compiled with the assistance of hundreds of brand-name manufacturers. Other sources are listed on page 61.

HarperCollins Publishers
Westerhill Road, Bishopbriggs, Glasgow G64 2QT

www.collins.co.uk

First published 2006

Reprint 10 9 8 7 6 5 4 3 2 1 0

© HarperCollins Publishers 2006

ISBN 0 00 722214-9

All rights reserved. Collins Gem® is a registered trademark of HarperCollinsPublishers Limited

Editorial by Grapevine Publishing Services, London
Text by Kate Santon
Design by Judith Ash

Printed in Italy by RotoLito

CONTENTS

INTRODUCTION

The ideal diet, from any dieter's point of view, is one that does not leave you feeling starved and deprived, and does not require perpetual weighing, measuring and calculating. Most importantly, it should enable you to lose excess weight and keep it off.

Recently all these claims have been made for the GI – glycaemic index – diets. A lot of people who have followed them have successfully reached their target weight, but the use of the GI diet in everyday life has also highlighted some problems and discrepancies. These have led to further refinements, and this is where the GL – glycaemic load – diet comes in.

In past decades, many other diets have gained swift popularity and it might seem as though the GI diet, and now the GL diets which have developed out of it, are following the same pattern. In reality, though, they are quite different from their predecessors. Here's a brief overview of some of the most popular diets and the weight-loss problems they address.

Many diets traditionally worked by restricting the intake of certain food groups or categories and substituting others; some simply restricted overall food intake. The problem with these restrictive diets is that

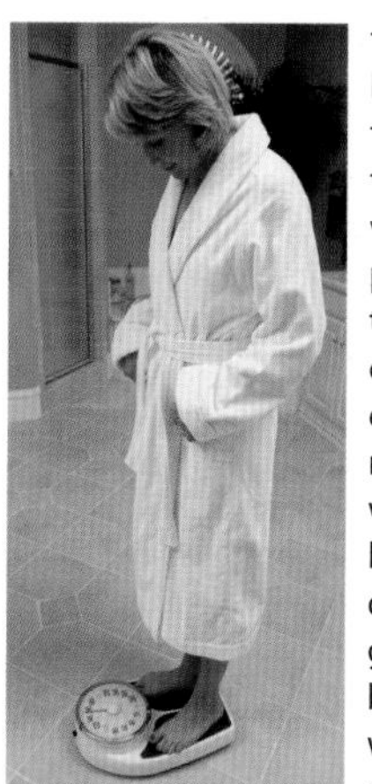

they left dieters feeling hungry, and also frequently tired, unfit and unwell. When they stopped dieting any weight they had lost just piled back on. They would then move on to another diet, which also failed in the end, and they didn't even manage to lose all the weight they'd regained. This led to a process of yo-yo dieting and gradual weight gain, something which is bad both for the metabolism as well as for self-respect and motivation. Repeated dieting does not make you thinner; it makes you fatter because your metabolism slows down.

There are dozens of bizarre, curiously restrictive diet ideas on the market; for example, those – like the Grapefruit Diet – on which you are only allowed to eat one type of food. There are meal-replacement diets and any number of strange, celebrity-endorsed eating plans. The only thing they have in common is that they don't work; fortunately most people get bored and give up before suffering any serious nutritional deficiencies.

Simple calorie counting diets are based on the premise that you gain weight if you take in more energy in food than you expend in exercise. Dieters cut back the calories they consume to sometimes very low levels – 1000 a day is not uncommon. Not only will they soon feel hungry and become bored with all the calculating, but reducing calorie intake to such levels affects the metabolism. Again, it is very difficult for calorie-counters to keep the weight off once they return to 'normal' patterns of eating and, because of the metabolic response, difficult for them to lose the weight they put back on.

There have also been diets targeting particular groups of foods. The *Atkins Diet* first made an impact in the 1970s when Dr Atkins publicised his idea that cutting out carbohydrates – bread, pasta, potatoes, most fruit and vegetables – would lead to weight loss. Atkins dieters concentrated on eating protein, especially foods high in fat, and many of them did lose weight. They also

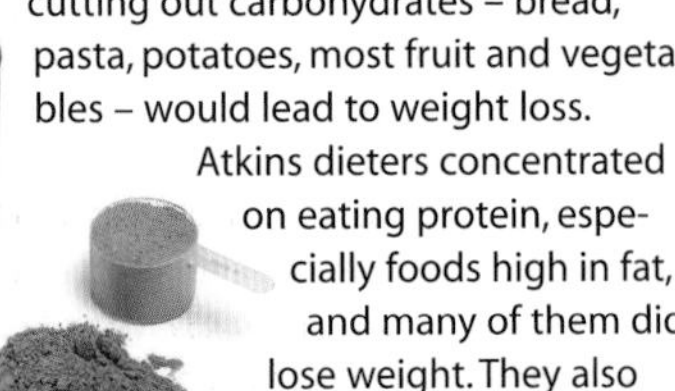

began suffering from severe constipation and bad breath. To deal with their problems, along came the *F Plan Diet*, developed by Audrey Eyton, which included fibre, lots of it, with every meal. Hunger was not a problem, and nor was constipation – the down-side was evident, however, by it being rechristened 'The Flatulence Plan'.

In the 1980s and early 90s fat was Rosemary Conley's enemy. However, the body actually needs some fat in order to function, and the fat in food also contributes to the level of satisfaction felt after eating. Dieters following her plans became exceptionally hungry and most gave up in the end.

Food combining, originally known as the *Hay Diet* and developed further by Harvey and Marilyn Diamond, was another option. Dieters were allowed to eat protein and carbohydrates, but not at the same meal. It could be difficult to follow in real life and most food combiners gave up; once they did, they gained weight again.

In the late 1990s and early years of the 21st century, with the government becoming more concerned about increasing obesity levels, new diets seemed to appear almost every week. Almost all of these began by pointing out where the previous bestseller had gone wrong, and many sprang into existence with little sound nutritional evidence to back them up. Some were punishingly severe, some were complex, some were a return to ancient principles of diet. The problems were the same, though; people became hungry, tired, unhealthy or bored, or found the diets difficult to follow, and when they gave up, whether they'd got to target or not, the weight they'd lost just reappeared.

At the end of the 1990s the *Atkins Diet* began a new surge in popularity, this time in a modified form permitting the consumption of some non-starchy carbs, though it still concentrated on proteins. Products like special low-carb bread were launched to help Atkins dieters stay on the straight and narrow, though the diet still relied on an induction phase in which carbs were cut out completely. When you do this your body burns fat for the fuel it needs and enters a state known as ketosis about which many doctors had severe reservations. Dieters going through ketosis suffered severe bad breath, constipation and a general feeling of ill health; some reported headaches, confusion and dizziness. A few deaths were alleged to have been caused by the diet, after the victims suffered severe metabolic imbalances, and there was

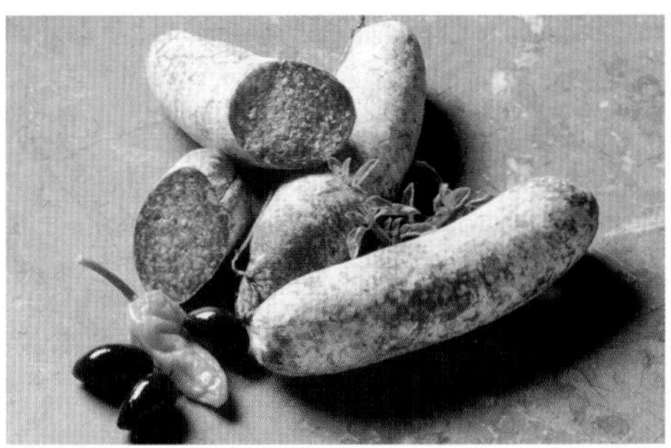

a lot of adverse publicity. Atkins Nutritionals has now filed for bankruptcy in the US. However, many Atkins dieters did lose weight, often very quickly and dramatically. Despite the problems, something interesting seemed to be happening. Whatever it was, when they stopped the diet the weight piled back on.

At about the same time, another diet began to attract attention. It didn't get the same level of publicity as Atkins but it seemed to be working for some people, who reported successful weight loss without feeling hungry, and they spread the word. The diet's creator, Michel Montignac, was already a bestselling author in France and, when his books were translated, he gained a wider audience. His 'Montignac

Method' wasn't easy to pigeonhole. It seemed to advocate that food from all groups could be eaten, but it wasn't strictly a food combining diet; in actual fact it drew on the relatively new knowledge of carbohydrates' glycaemic index. This had also started to feature in a few other plans, such as the *South Beach Diet*, as people began to realise that the key to weight loss might lie in using the body's natural responses and regulating blood sugar levels.

BLOOD SUGAR

During digestion, the starch in carbohydrates – there is a lot of it in potatoes, cereals, bread and pasta – becomes glucose, a sugar which the body uses as an energy source. Glucose enters the bloodstream rapidly and the overall level of sugar in the blood shoots up, causing a blood sugar 'spike'. This prompts the pancreas to produce high quantities of the hormone insulin to deal with the excessive sugar

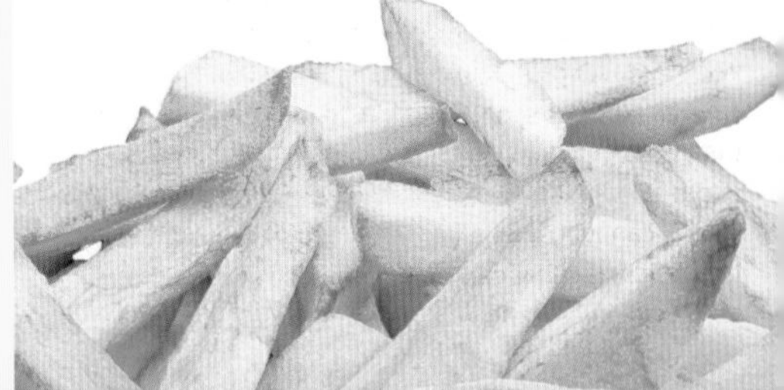

levels. Insulin helps glucose to enter the cells of the body to become available as energy; the problem for anyone trying to lose weight is that it also inhibits the release of stored fat.

Another related problem is that high glucose levels drop away very fast as the extra insulin does its job. This fall signals your body to boost the glucose level again – and you end up feeling hungrier than ever, and possibly reaching for a biscuit to deal with the pangs. So keeping insulin levels steady is vital if you're trying to lose weight – and to do that you have to stabilise your blood sugar levels.

Diabetics and dieters

People with diabetes know all about the importance of keeping blood sugar – and therefore insulin – levels as steady as possible. There are two kinds of diabetes. In both types, sufferers fail to produce enough insulin, but those with type 2 diabetes develop the condition later in life and can often control it with diet, or with a combination of diet and medication. Type 1 diabetes sufferers are dependent on insulin injections. For both groups, controlling blood sugar is critical; if they don't, they risk a diabetic crisis which can lead to a coma and is fatal if untreated. Diabetics used to be advised to eat lots of starchy carbs, but this was problematic because such carbs release their sugar into the bloodstream quickly. Blood sugar spikes can lead to possible collapse, so it was important to learn more about this. Gradually researchers found that not all carbs produced spikes; some were broken down more slowly than others and controlled scientific trials showed that it was far better for diabetics to eat carbs that were less disruptive. As an added benefit, this seemed to smooth out the level of blood sugar over the day.

Researchers in several centres worldwide began to develop the glycaemic index (GI) of carbohydrates, as a reference point for comparing different foods. This was followed by the GL – glycaemic load – which modified some of the GI's shortcomings. Scientific trials with diabetics showed that eating a low-GI diet significantly improved blood sugar control and the idea of using the GI to control weight began to spread outside the diabetic community.

HOW DO GI AND GL WORK?

Scientists gave scores to the different types of carbs they were testing, according to how fast they were converted into blood sugar. Glucose itself (or sometimes white bread) was the control, with a glycaemic index score of 100. A food with a low GI (under 55)

The Glucose Process

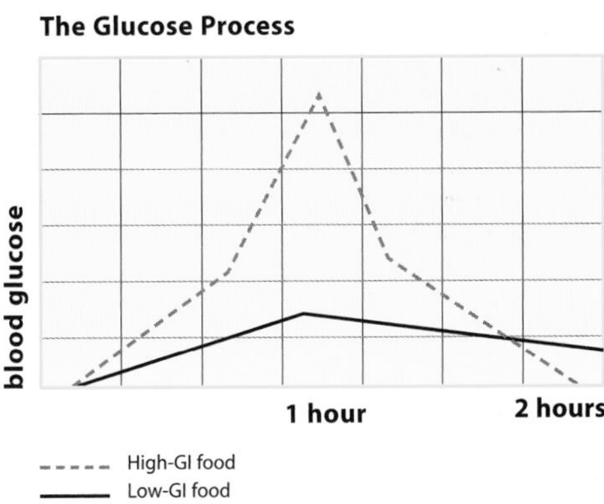

breaks down slowly, giving a slow rise in blood sugar and insulin levels, whereas foods with high GI levels – like white flour – break down much more quickly and send blood sugar and insulin levels soaring.

But it wasn't as simple as that; there were strange inconsistencies which stemmed from the way food was being tested. Ten or more healthy people were given a precise measure of the food in question first thing in the morning. This measure usually consisted of whatever portion size contains 50g of carbs, so that the rises in blood sugar levels caused by different foods could be compared like for like. The human guinea pigs had their blood sugar levels monitored at specific intervals over the next two hours and the results were averaged and used to plot a curve on a graph. This curve was then compared with the reference food – usually glucose – which is given a value of 100.

One problem became clear quite quickly. GI values failed to take into account actual portion sizes. To get 50g-worth of carbs in white sugar you'd need relatively little, but to get the same carb content from something like broccoli you'd need more. A lot more: a test portion of broccoli – one containing 50g of carbohydrate – would weigh about 5kg! So, because the GI in isolation can sometimes be misleading, another measurement has been developed – the GL.

The glycaemic load of a food is calculated by multiplying its GI value by the number of grams of carb contained in a realistic portion, and then dividing the result by 100.

GI value x grams of carb per serving ÷ 100 = GL value

GL values are much lower than those of the GI. High GI foods have a value of 70 or more; medium ones are in the 56–69 range, and low ones are those at 55 and below. A food with a high GL has a value of 20 or more, one with a medium GL falls in the 11–19 range, and a low GL food would have a value of 10 or less.

In the cases of both GI and GL, foods are usually just designated high, medium or low, and given a red, yellow or green traffic-light coding. Giving specific values to each food could never be entirely accurate, because you will find slight variations in GI and GL from one kind of apple to the next, or from one slice of bread to the next. That's why foods are often categorised within a range.

Once portion size is taken into consideration the discrepancies become clearer. Some foods that are particularly carbohydrate-dense, like pasta, can substantially increase blood sugar and insulin levels if enough is eaten, so they have a high GL. And 'enough' need not be a huge amount, either. Even though pasta generally has a low or medium GI depending on the type, just two cups of cooked macaroni or spaghetti have a high GL.

This also works in reverse. Some foods which have a high GI actually have a low GL once portion sizes are taken into account. Consider the following:

Cantaloupe melon	GI value 65	GL value 3
Watermelon	GI value 72	GL value 6
Pumpkin	GI value 75	GL value 1
Broad beans, cooked	GI value 80	GL value 18

There are others. Carrots are often cited; they have a medium GI but a low GL, and many purely GI diets advise that you cut them out. There really is no need to do so.

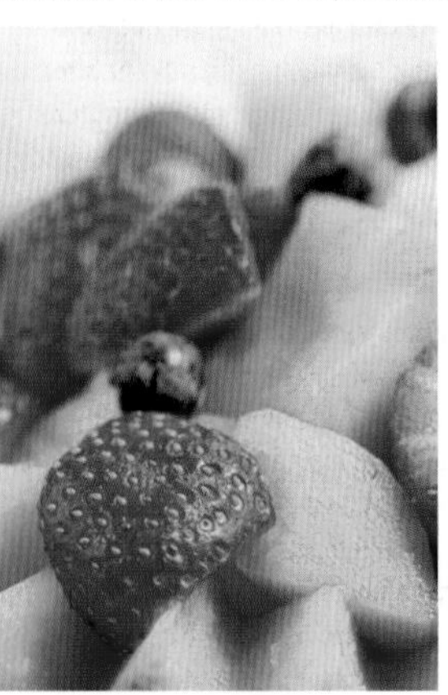

So GL or GI?

The GL considers quantity as well as quality, but in major studies at Harvard University it has been found to work best in tandem with some consideration of the GI. The overall GI value of a subject's diet can be a tool for predicting their risk of getting certain diseases and can give a good indication of their general health. Much that applies to a GI diet also applies to a GL diet, because one is derived from the other. The GL identifies the exceptions to the GI, but the same broad principles apply to both. However, the GL reflects the actual effect the carb you are eating will have on your body, and dieters may find it easier to use in practice because it regulates your blood sugar levels more carefully.

This does not mean that every low-GL, or even low GI, food will help you to lose weight. Other factors have to be considered. White bread and wholemeal bread have similar GL values, but one will add nutritional value to your diet – wholemeal contains many more nutrients and fibre – and one will not. Also, a food only has a GI/GL value if it contains carbs, and lots of foods which are high in calories – like butter or full-fat cream – have none.

You can't rely on GL values in isolation if you want to lose weight; eating huge amounts of protein and fat will not make you slimmer or healthier. Let common sense be your guide; for example, smothering spinach (low GL) in butter (no GL) will not help with weight loss, however low the overall GL.

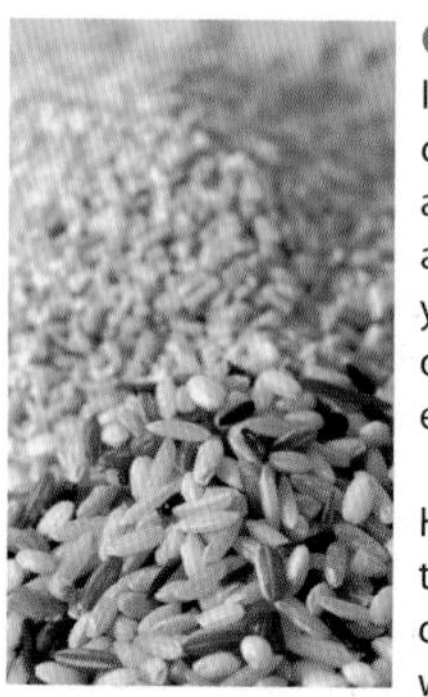

Carbs to choose

It's not always obvious which carbs are high GL and which are low, but fortunately there are a couple of guidelines you can use to help you decide what you should be eating.

How sweet is it? The sweeter the taste of a food, the more quickly your blood sugar level will rise when you eat it. Sugars – sometimes called simple carbohydrates – are the carbs that affect your blood sugar the fastest.

Fibre is a also a good guide, and packaged foods will all have their fibre count listed on the ingredients label. The amount of fibre in whole grains, beans, seeds, pulses and some vegetables means that they are digested much more slowly than their refined equivalents. They need to be broken down and therefore take more time to be absorbed into the bloodstream, leading to a gentler rise in blood sugar levels. The manufacturing processes used to refine some foods – like rice (which is treated to make it quicker to cook), white flour, biscuits, ready meals and cakes – remove a lot of their fibre content, so they are converted into glucose very quickly compared to their unrefined equivalent.

Some GL diet rules

- Don't skip meals. You're supposed to eat on the GL diet, not avoid eating. If you miss meals your blood sugar levels will drop and the aim is to keep them steady.

- Carbs with a tougher coat, like whole grains, take longer for your body to digest and therefore take longer to cause rises in blood sugar. So if a food – even a wholegrain food – is ground, mashed, puréed, peeled or otherwise processed, it will be much more easily broken down into glucose. Wholemeal bread, for example, has a lower GL if it has some seeds and whole grains on top. A creamy, smooth vegetable soup will be digested much more quickly than its raw vegetable ingredients, or even just a rougher version of the same soup. A whole fruit or vegetable is better than its juice – there's much more fibre in a whole orange than there is in orange juice.

- Cooking can also have an effect on GL values. The longer a vegetable is boiled, for instance, the less fibre it retains. So cooking vegetables quickly and eating them while they still have some crunch is better. (Over-boiling also reduces the amount of nutrients they contain.) Steaming or quickly stir-frying are two of the best methods.

- Some starches are more easily broken down than others. Brown basmati rice isn't just higher in fibre than the glutinous white rice served in a Thai restaurant; it also contains a starch called amylose, which is less easily digested. If the granules of starch have swollen and burst, then the rice will be digested speedily. However, don't forget that all kinds of rice have a high GL so shouldn't be part of the weight-loss phase of a GL diet plan.

- While you have to be careful with fats because they are high-calorie, they can slow down the digestion of carbs, reducing the effects of higher-GL food on blood sugar. Proteins have the same effect, so look at your meal as a whole. You can moderate the effects of a high-GL food by being selective about what you eat with it.

- One of the more recently appreciated effects of acids is that sprinkling lemon juice or vinegar over your food can reduce overall GL. So a little lemon juice over a salad containing pasta is a good idea.

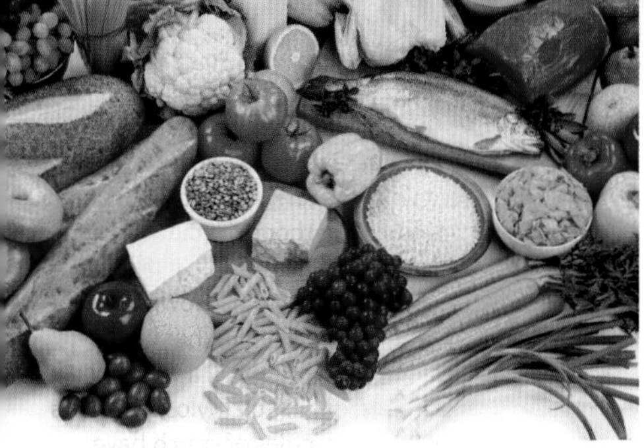

- Once again, remember that the GL index only measures the effects of carbs; it doesn't measure calories, so don't go wild with no-GL food. Remember also that the GL of a food is dependent on the portion size. Large helpings will push GL levels way up and undermine your diet.

- One more food item to consider is sugar. It might be the first thing you think of cutting out when you diet – the phrase 'empty calories' is often used – but on the GL diet it doesn't have to be omitted completely. Once again, portion control is vital, so you need to be strong-willed. If you follow up all the healthy food you are eating with a high-sugar dessert or snack, you'll undo all your positive efforts. Think about the sugar content of each food you buy and check labels carefully; it is very easy to increase your overall intake without even noticing. In addition sugar can be addictive; if you can keep to a little, give it a try. If you know you won't be able to stop at the odd teaspoon, you might be better off cutting sugar out. Try weaning yourself off it gradually if that's hard.

The Food Pyramid

If you follow all the GL guidelines properly, you'll be well on the way to eating a balanced diet. This is one of the reasons why medical professionals are in favour of it and is one of the GI and GL diets' major advantages over the more restrictive, faddy diets that flit in and out of fashion. A diet that excludes whole food groups like fats or carbs does your health no good at all – and may even cause you harm – and it won't help you to keep excess weight off for good.

The GL diet gives you all the nutrients your body needs. The food groups should be in the right proportions relative to each other, but this is not hard to achieve. The GL food pyramid (*opposite*) is a representation of the different food groups and the number of portions you should eat of each on a daily basis.

- Vegetables and fruit (but not potatoes): 5–8 portions a day

- Grains, cereals, potatoes, pasta, rice: 2–3 portions a day. Choose low-GL varieties like rye or pumpernickel bread, porridge or muesli, and go easy on potatoes, pasta and especially rice.
- Dairy products: 1–3 portions a day. Remember that some of these can be very high in calories. Choose skimmed milk and low- or no-fat options.
- Proteins (lean meat, fish, poultry, eggs, beans, tofu and nuts): 1–3 portions a day.

The GL Food Pyramid

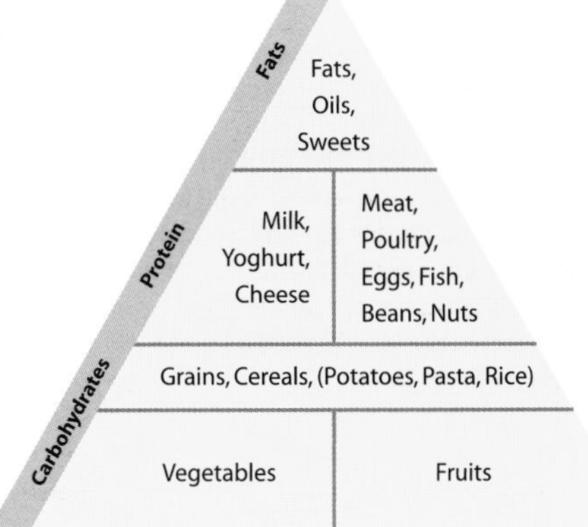

- Fats and oils: use in moderation for cooking or for salad dressings. See page 33 for the healthiest types.

Portion control

Never pile your plate with huge servings; that blows the whole GL diet theory wide open. Choosing the correct portion sizes is important, but you don't need to weigh and measure if you follow the guidelines below.

Bakery

In the weight-loss phase, limit yourself to 2 slices of low-GL bread a day at most. A medium slice of bread is one that weighs around 30g.

Beans and Pulses

A portion is about half a teacup of cooked beans or drained canned beans, and will weigh about 115g. Note that a small can of beans in sauce weighs 200g – but these should be avoided as they almost certainly contain too much sugar.

Breakfast cereals

A portion of bran cereal (40g) or muesli (50g) will fill about half an average-sized bowl; 30g dry weight porridge oats is slightly less than half a normal bowl and makes a good helping when cooked.

Condiments and Sauces
15ml is a level tablespoon and 5ml is a level teaspoon. Use a medicine spoon as a 5ml measure.

Meat and Poultry
A 75g piece of meat or chicken is about the same size as a pocket pack of tissues. A100g piece is roughly the size of a pack of cards.

Pasta
There's no easy visual measure as pasta shapes vary, so this is best weighed. Eat rarely, choose wholemeal and don't, in general, have more than 50g dry weight, which will be approximately 100g when cooked.

Rice
Rice has a very high GL and should be avoided during the weight-loss phase of your diet. 2 level tablespoons of dry rice makes about 75g when cooked – a mound roughly the same size as a woman's fist.

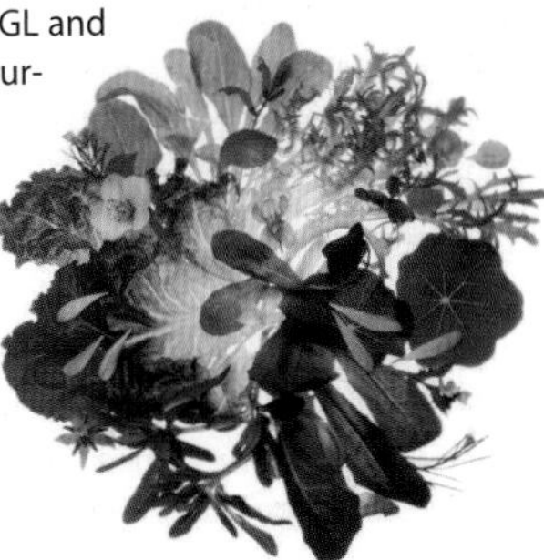

Snacks
25g nuts is roughly the amount a small child could hold in one hand.

Sugar and honey
Stick to 1 tsp a day (level, not rounded).

Vegetables
Most of the portion sizes given in the listings are equivalent to half a teacupful, unless otherwise stated. A teacup of salad leaves weighs about 30g.
Half a cup of cooked shredded cabbage is roughly 75g.

There's another simple guide to portion control: your plate. Divide it mentally into quarters. Two of these should be filled with vegetables, one quarter with protein, and one quarter with another carb – a few baby new potatoes, or a small helping of pasta perhaps. Choose the lowest-GL carb you can – so 2–3 new potatoes rather than mash, wholemeal pasta rather than ordinary white pasta.

Be reasonable. Use a normal dinner plate, not a huge platter. Don't pile the food up high just to fit it on to a quarter of the surface area. After a while you'll discover that it's easy to be sensible on the GL diet as hunger isn't a problem.

WHAT KIND OF PROTEINS AND FATS?

There are two main types of dietary fat – saturated and unsaturated. Saturated fats tend to come from animal protein sources: the white fat on cuts of meat, butter, cream and cheese, lard or dripping. Unsaturated fats include vegetable, fish and nut oils.

Proteins are essential for good health, providing the materials from which bones, muscles, hair, nails, blood, enzymes and hormones are created.

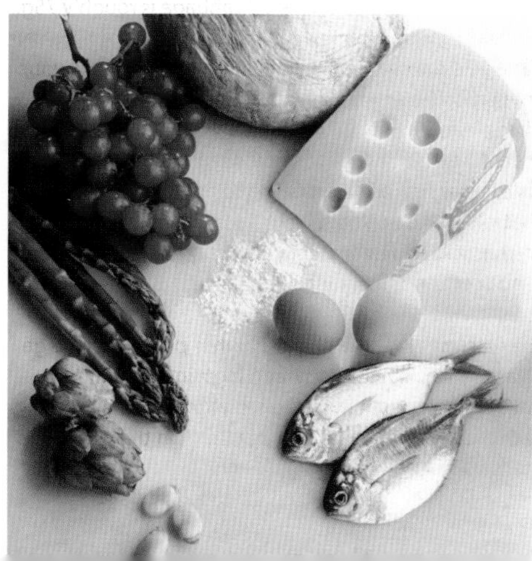

They aren't just found in meat, fish, cheese and eggs, though; vegetable proteins include soya products like tofu, beans and pulses, brown rice, broccoli, bananas and many other fruits and vegetables. Adults only need 60g of protein a day, but most of us eat a lot more.

As most people will be aware, saturated fats (from animal sources) got a bad name because they became associated with high levels of cholesterol blocking the arteries and triggering heart disease and stroke. However, Atkins diets advocate eating full-fat proteins, because they make you feel fuller and add flavour to food while slowing the absorption of carbs. The Atkins research centres claim that people following their diet show a reduction in blood pressure and improved cholesterol levels. However, most medical professionals and certainly the vast majority of heart specialists give the opposite advice – that you should choose low-fat or fat-free dairy products and lean meats – and most GL diets go along with the low-fat approach.

Having said that, we all need some fats in our diet, even when trying to lose weight, because important nutrients are supplied by 'good' fats. The following tells you which fats to opt for and which to avoid:

- Monounsaturated fats, found in olive and rapeseed oil, walnuts and almonds, have beneficial effects on the heart.

- Omega 3 fats, found in oily fishes like salmon, mackerel and herring, flaxseed oils, wheatgerm and soya beans, help to thin the blood and are crucial for brain function.

- Polyunsaturated fats, found in vegetable and corn oils, don't have the health benefits of mono-unsaturated fats but, like most fats, they contain 135 calories per tablespoonful, so should be used sparingly when you're trying to lose weight.

- Saturated fats include all the animal fats, plus coconut and palm oils, which are often

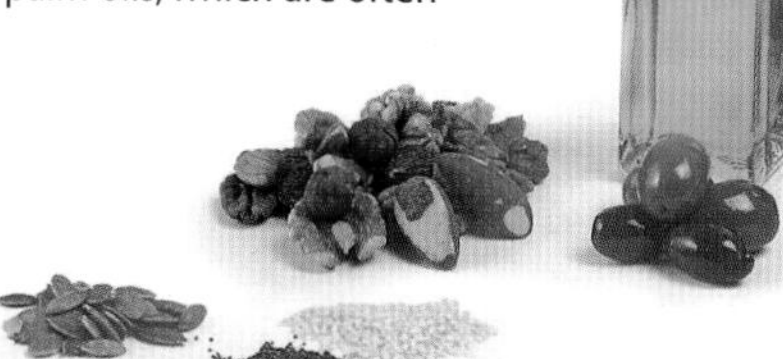

found in biscuits and snacks. Try to avoid eating them too frequently.

- Hydrogenated or trans fats are the worst type, linked to high cholesterol levels and increased heart disease risk. You'll find them in various kinds of ready-made meals, biscuits and cakes, breads and spreads, vegetable shortening, peanut butter, pastries, margarines and fast foods.

VITAMINS AND MINERALS

On paper, GL diets are healthy, but in practice it's up to each individual to make sure they eat a wide enough range of foods to get all the vitamins and minerals they need for good health. One tip is to make sure all the fruits and vegetables you eat in a day are different colours: dark green kale, yellow corn, red peppers, orange carrots, translucent onions, pale green avocados, pale yellow melon, purple sprouting broccoli, blackberries, apricots, blueberries, bananas. Your meals will look more attractive, and you will be getting different types of micronutrient from each.

Try to make sure that you eat foods containing each of the following vitamins and minerals on a daily – or at least weekly – basis.

Vitamin A: eggs, butter, fish oils, dark green and yellow fruits and vegetables, liver.
Essential for: strong bones, good eyesight, healthy skin, healing.

Vitamin B1 (*Thiamine*): plant and animal foods, especially wholegrain products, brown rice, seafood and beans.
Essential for: growth, nerve function, conversion of blood sugar into energy.

Vitamin B2 (*Riboflavin*): Milk and dairy produce, green leafy vegetables, liver, kidneys, yeast.
Essential for: cell growth and reproduction, energy production.

Vitamin B3 (*Niacin*): meats, fish and poultry, wholegrains, peanuts and avocados.
Essential for: digestion, energy, the nervous system.

Vitamin B5 (*Pantothenic acid*): organ meats, fish, eggs, chicken, nuts and wholegrain cereals.
Essential for: strengthening immunity and fighting infections, healing wounds.

Vitamin B6 (*Pyridoxine*): meat, eggs, wholegrains, yeast, cabbage, melon, molasses.
Essential for: the production of new cells, a healthy immune system, production of

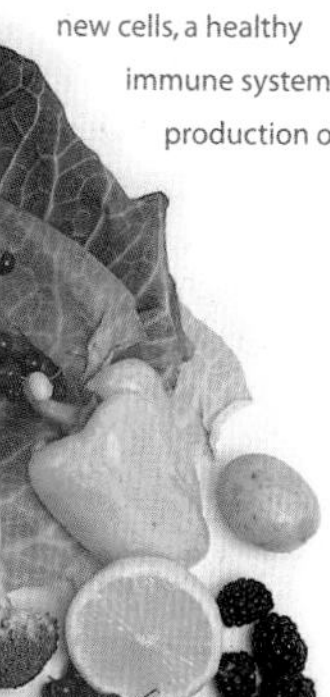

antibodies and white blood cells.

Vitamin B12 (*Cyanocobalamin*): fish, dairy produce, beef, pork, lamb, organ meats, eggs and milk.

Essential for: energy and concentration, production of red blood cells, growth in children.

Vitamin C: fresh fruit and vegetables, potatoes, leafy herbs and berries.

Essential for: healthy skin, bones, muscles, healing, eyesight and protection from viruses.

Vitamin D: milk and dairy produce, eggs, fatty fish.

Essential for: healthy teeth and bones, vital for growth.

Vitamin E: nuts, seeds, eggs, milk, wholegrains, leafy green vegetables, avocados and soya.

Essential for: absorption of iron and essential fatty acids, slowing the ageing process, increasing fertility.

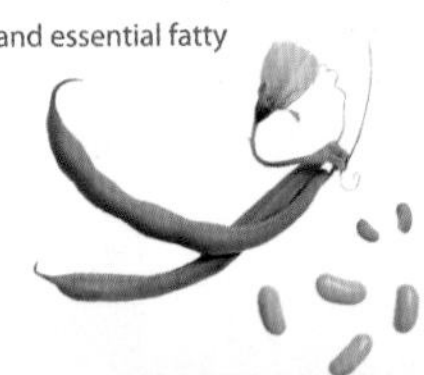

Vitamin K: green vegetables, milk products, apricots, wholegrains, cod liver oil.

Essential for: blood clotting.

Calcium: dairy produce, leafy green vegetables, salmon, nuts, root vegetables, tofu.

Essential for: strong bones and teeth, hormones and muscles, blood clotting and the regulation of blood pressure.

Iron: liver, kidney, cocoa powder, dark chocolate, shellfish, pulses, dark green vegetables, egg yolks, red meat, beans, molasses.

Essential for: supply of oxygen to the cells and healthy immune system.

Magnesium: brown rice, soya beans, nuts, wholegrains, bitter chocolate, legumes.

Essential for: transmission of nerve impulses, development of bones, growth and repair of cells.

Potassium: avocados, leafy green vegetables, bananas, fruit and vegetable juices, potatoes and nuts.
Essential for: maintaining water balance, nerve and muscle function.

Chromium: liver, wholegrains, meat and cheese, brewer's yeast, mushrooms, egg yolk.
Essential for: stimulating insulin. Chromium also governs the 'glucose tolerance factor' which is often not working properly in failed dieters.

Iodine: fish and seafood, pineapple, dairy produce, raisins.
Essential for: keeping hair, skin, nails and teeth healthy.

Folic acid: fruit, green leafy vegetables, nuts, pulses, yeast extracts.
Essential for: production of new cells (working with vitamin B12) and especially important during pregnancy to help prevent birth defects.

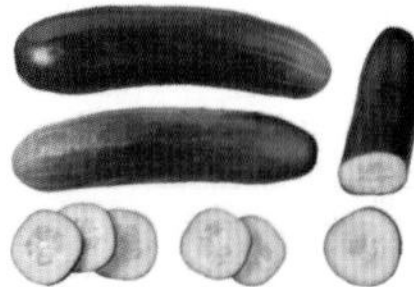

SUPPLEMENTS

If you are unable to get all the vitamins and minerals you need from fresh food, you should consider taking a supplement, but never exceed the Recommended Daily Allowance (RDA) as indicated on the pack, because some can be dangerous in high doses. Alternatively, look out for foods that have vitamins and minerals added. The packaging should indicate the percentage of the RDA they supply.

READING LABELS

You won't find GL values listed on the packaging of many foods in the UK, although Tesco have introduced a rated GI logo for some of their own-brand foods, which can be useful. However, reading the ingredients labels and bearing in mind the basic GL rules outlined above should help you to make an informed decision about which foods are low GL. Ingredients are listed on food packaging in descending order of volume, so if sugars or fats are near the beginning, alarm bells should start ringing.

- Watch out for sugar in all its guises: it might be labelled glucose, sucrose, invertase, fructose, lactose, galactose, maltose, dextrose or honey.

- You will probably recognise the names for fats. Watch out for hydrogenated, partially hydrogenated or trans fats, and give them a wide berth.

- Long lists of E numbers, artificial colours and flavours are always a turn-off.

Under Nutrition Information, look for the following:

- Calorie count should be given per portion, per pack and/or per 100g or 100ml serving. Note that manufacturers' portion sizes can be extremely small and it can be easy to eat twice as much as they estimate. Don't overlook calories on a low-GL diet – you will put on weight if you are consuming more calories a day than you are burning off through exercise, regardless of whether they are 'low-GL' calories.

- Carbohydrates will be listed, and the label will probably indicate how much of the carb total is made up of sugars. The more sugars, the more quickly it could affect your blood sugar level.

- Fat content will be given as total fat, then the percentage of saturates, monounsaturates and polyunsaturates will be listed. Remember to opt for monounsaturates if possible.

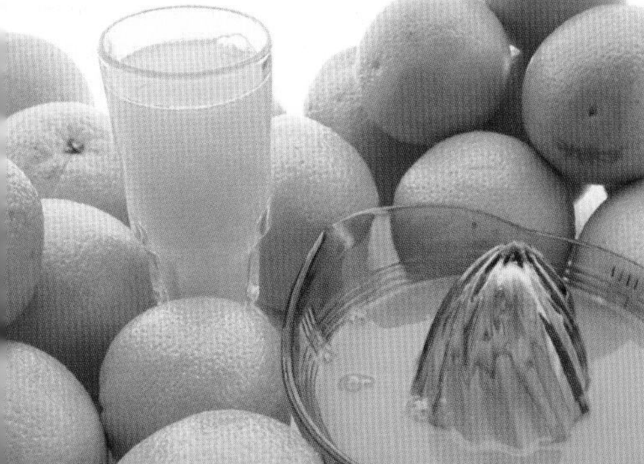

- Choose high-fibre products; aim for more than 5g fibre per 100g serving.

- Are there vitamins and minerals listed? The percentage of the Recommended Daily Allowance supplied by an average portion or per 100g/100ml should be given.

Nutrition flashes on the front of packaging can be misleading:

- The term 'fat-free' can be applied to foods containing less than 0.15g fat per 100g. However, the term '90% fat-free' means that the product actually has 10% fat.

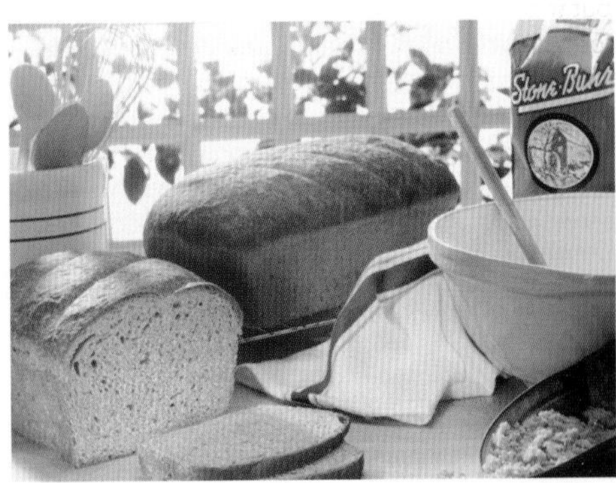

- 'Virtually fat-free' means the food contains less than 0.3g fat per 100g. 'Low-fat' means the food must contain 3g or fewer of fat per 100g. 'Reduced fat' means the food contains 25% less fat than the standard equivalent product.

- 'No added sugar' means that no sugar has been added during processing or manufacture but it does not necessarily mean that the food is low in sugar. 'Unsweetened' means that no sugar or sweetener has been added.

- There is no legal definition of the term 'reduced salt' but the Food Standards Agency recommends that food with this label should contain 25% less salt or sodium than an equivalent product.

- 'Rich source of...' a vitamin or mineral means the product must contain 50% of the RDA in a typical serving. If it says 'Source of...' then a serving must contain at least 17% of the RDA.

HOW MUCH WEIGHT DO YOU NEED TO LOSE?

Before you start any weight-loss diet, you should have an idea of what would be a healthy weight for you. There's no point in setting unrealistic goals. If you have a naturally rounded figure, you will make yourself ill trying to diet down to stick-insect proportions. If you have a large frame, you will never shrink to a small frame no matter how little you eat. Everyone is born with a genetically predisposed natural weight range. If you consistently eat too much and don't exercise, your weight will exceed this range. If you diet down to a weight below your natural range, you will find it hard to maintain.

Height and weight charts are just approximations that reflect cultural averages. Two people of the same height and build can have completely different weights and yet both be healthy. Muscle weighs more than fat, so someone who exercises regularly might weigh more than someone of the same height who is sedentary. This is why doctors are now more likely to calculate your body mass index (BMI) to see whether you are overweight or not. BMI is a height to weight formula that gives a good approximation of the quantity of total body fat you are carrying. To find your BMI, divide your weight in kilograms by the square of your height in metres:

weight ÷ (height x height)

For example, if you are 1.75m tall and weigh 64kg:

1.75 x 1.75 = 3.06
64 ÷ 3.06 = 20.91

Check your total against the list below to see if you fall into an average range.

less than 15	emaciated
15–19	underweight
19–25	average
25–30	overweight
30–40	obese

If your BMI is in the emaciated or obese range, you should consult your doctor for advice, as you could be seriously endangering your health.

WAIST MEASUREMENT

Waist measurements of more than 100cm (40 inches) for men and more than 88cm (35 inches) for women are linked with all kinds of health risks, particularly an increased risk of heart disease. Another indicator that doctors use is your waist to hip ratio:

waist measurement ÷ hip measurement = ?

Above 1.0 for men and 0.85 for women puts you into an at-risk category.

Your ideal weight is generally the one at which you feel healthy, energetic and comfortable. Once you reach an 'average' BMI score, then you are a healthy weight. Ask yourself, how much do you think you want to lose? What BMI rating would this give for your height? So how much do you need to lose to take you down into an average BMI category? This is a sensible target to aim for.

Don't try to lose more than a kilogram a week, or you will be likely to put it all back on again as soon as you stop dieting. Slow and steady is the best plan. If you want to lose 10 kilos, allow at least three months; for

WARNING

Consult a doctor before starting a weight-loss programme if:

- you have a chronic condition such as coronary heart disease, or have had a stroke
- you take any medication
- you are pregnant
- you are over 40 and have more than 5 kilos to lose
- you are planning to start an exercise programme as well, but haven't exercised for years.

20 kilos, allow at least 6 months; and for 40 kilos, give yourself a year. A realistic target is to lose between 5 and 10% of your starting weight within 6 months.

EXERCISE

Most weight-loss experts agree that the first thing you should do on a diet plan is to increase your level of physical activity. Muscle burns more calories than fat, so once you increase the amount of muscle in your body, you will be burning off more energy even when you are sitting watching television.

No matter what kind of diet you decide to follow, calories still count. To lose half a kilo per week, you need to reduce your calorie intake by 500 kcal a day or 3,500 per week. However, a one-hour aerobics class might burn off around 400 kcal; half an hour of jogging could burn 250 kcal, and 15 minutes of brisk walking could burn 75 kcal. This means that if you are exercising, you won't need to cut back on what you eat quite so drastically!

There is also evidence to suggest that exercise helps to keep your blood sugar levels steady by triggering the release of hormones that regulate them. It also stimulates the release of endorphins, which make you feel good and relieve stress and depression.

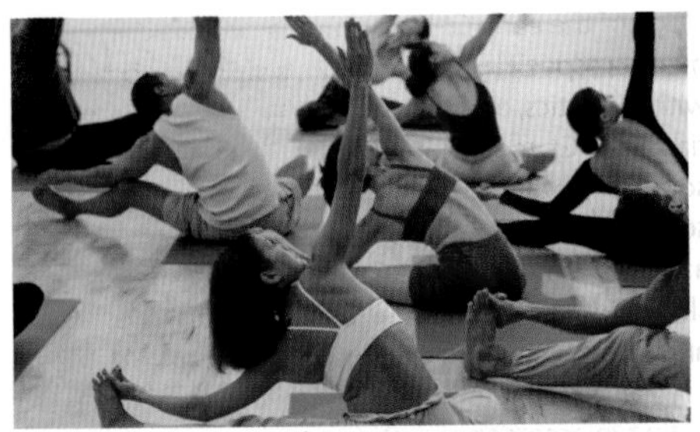

You'll see results much faster if you combine your GL diet with a new exercise or weight-loss plan, which will help to keep you motivated – which means you'll reach your target weight more quickly. And with any luck, you'll keep your exercise habit for life.

WHY CHOOSE A GL DIET?

The GL diet isn't a fad diet, nor is it short term. It is essentially a method of applying healthy eating principles and using the way your body works naturally in order to lose weight – and then to maintain that weight loss. It doesn't involve cutting out any type of food that your body needs in order to function and it's not going to make you ill. For all these reasons the medical establishment, from the World Health Organisation (WHO) downwards, approve of GI/GL.

Many of the early GI-based diets were developed by medics, especially cardiologists and those working with diabetics, or by scientists and qualified dietitians. The GL modifications came from similarly sound scientific research. All of this could make it sound as though it was going to be fiddly, requiring a deep scientific knowledge and advanced maths skills, but it doesn't – it's easy. It's also sustainable, and one of the reasons for that is that it's enjoyable.

Eating in accordance with GI and GL guidelines is something that can – and as the WHO recommends, should – be done for the good of our health. It reduces the risk of developing type 2 diabetes, having a heart attack or stroke, and will also increase your energy levels.

In many ways it's a return to eating in the way we did before we all came to rely on processed food, ready meals and refined ingredients, but without spending hours and hours in the kitchen. It is easy to adapt quick and convenient recipes and you can freeze portions of your own home-cooked dishes for some healthy 'ready' meals.

You need to understand some basic nutrition to follow the GL diet, but it really is very little. As you cook and eat, this soon becomes second nature. You also have to keep an eye on portion sizes, but in a simple, straightforward way. Maintaining your weight after you've reached target is easy too, because you will have changed the way you eat. The GL diet isn't just a quick-fix campaign for a few weeks – it's a healthy eating plan for life. There are several GL diet books on the market, but here we look at two of the main ones and analyse how they work.

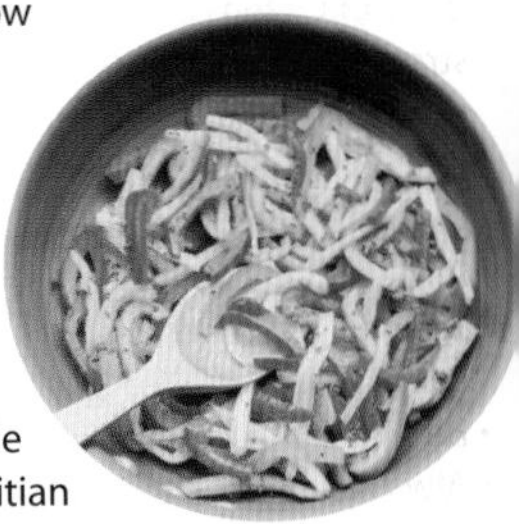

NIGEL DENBY'S *THE GL DIET*

Nigel Denby worked as a chef and restaurant owner before retraining as a registered dietitian. He worked as a research dietitian at the Human Nutrition Research Centre in Newcastle, and in the NHS, and is now a consultant working with bodies like the International Eating Disorders Centre and Hammersmith and Queen Charlotte's Hospital Women's Health Clinic. A reformed serial dieter, he originally began by applying the nutritional science he was studying to himself, and found that it worked as a practical way of losing weight.

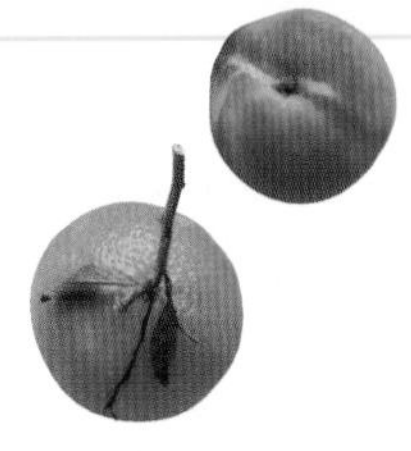

Denby stresses that eating in accordance with GL principles is a long-term, healthy lifestyle change. He suggests that before starting you keep a food diary recording what you eat and when, to identify particular areas that could prove problematic. He stresses the importance of both regular exercise and positive thinking.

Golden rules

- Aim to eat 3 meals a day.
- Try not to let more than 4 hours go by without eating something.
- Be flexible.
- Always have average-sized portions; don't super-size.
- Clear out any trigger foods that might lead you astray – like biscuits, sweets, chocolate.
- Move about more!

There are no phases to progress through (though there is some advice about introducing more food once your target weight has been reached) nor are there any menu plans. The idea is to improvise, choosing dishes to suit yourself and your circumstances. There are guidelines to follow to make sure that your diet is varied: eat lots of different coloured fruit and vegetables, plenty of fibre and a variety of protein-based foods, with small amounts of dairy. And the abundance of suggestions for meals and snacks, and extensive recipes, make this relatively easy to do. The same flexibility applies to other areas of the diet as well, such as monitoring weight loss, for example; it is up to you how often you weight yourself.

There are lists of suitable foods and advice on sensible shopping. Unlike many diet plans, this one offers advice on how to choose appropriate ready meals if necessary, though Denby does stress the importance of cooking as much of your food as possible yourself. The majority of the recipes are quick to prepare.

On this diet, desserts are really for special occasions, but low-GL fruit or yoghurt can be eaten every day if you need something sweet. Denby points out that you lose weight more easily if you avoid alcohol, but he adds that red wine is the best choice for anyone who finds that impossible. He suggests trying to wean yourself off sugar, using fructose if you find that difficult, and allows the 'odd teaspoonful' of honey as a substitute. There is plenty of information about how to make sensible choices when eating out.

Foods to enjoy	Foods to limit	Foods to avoid
Fresh fruit	Potatoes, other than baby new potatoes	Sugar in all its guises
Fresh vegetables	Some root vegetables, like parsnips	White bread
Fresh meat and fish	Dairy products, including cheese	Biscuits
Porridge oats, oat bran couscous	Pasta	Corn products, like tortilla chips, cornmeal and polenta
	Chocolate	Rice

Menu suggestions

Breakfast choices: Bacon and tomato omelette; muesli; two papaya halves with freshly squeezed lemon or lime juice.

Lunch choices: Carrot and coriander soup; mozzarella cheese and tomato slices with a balsamic dressing; smoked mackerel pâté on low-GL toast.

Dinner choices: chicken korma; peppered pork with chestnut mushrooms; vegetable kebabs with gado-gado sauce.

Snacks: Low-GL fruit or vegetable crudités; dried apricots; sunflower seeds.

Effectiveness

You need self-discipline to follow Nigel Denby's diet, which is effectively a change in your lifestyle. Providing you are sensible, there is no reason why you should not lose weight steadily, as the diet is practical and realistic. It is also simple to incorporate into

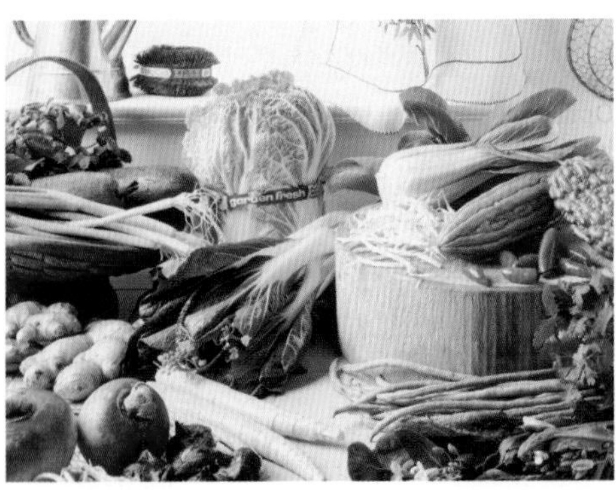

everyday life, and not too disruptive for family members; in fact, it can motivate everyone in the family to eat more healthily.

Vegetarians are well catered for, as well as meat-eaters; all the food recommended is familiar and easily available and the recipes are tasty. It will also appeal undoubtedly to those with an independent streak, who don't necessarily want to be told what they will be eating three weeks on Wednesday. Additional support, if needed, is available online (see Useful Websites, page 239).

PATRICK HOLFORD'S *THE HOLFORD DIET*

Patrick Holford, who founded the Institute for Optimum Nutrition in the 1980s, is one of Britain's leading nutritionists. Through personal experience, while studying psychology at York University, he discovered he impact of making radical changes to his diet on weight and overall health. His work with diet and nutrition since then has led to the development of *The Holford Diet*, and also a Holford Diet recipe book.

The diet is part of a larger programme which advocates eliminating any hidden allergies and taking a range of food supplements. He also recommends 15 minutes of exercise daily. The diet itself aims to control blood sugar levels and ensure that people following it eat only good fats.

Holford advises setting realistic targets, pointing out that many people begin a new diet hoping 'to lose in a week what they gained in a year'. Before beginning the initial phase, dieters are advised to prepare themselves the week beforehand by cutting out all stimulants – tea, coffee, alcohol, chocolate and cigarettes. None should be used while on the diet itself; red meat is also not included in the diet. This is the time to remove edible temptations and restock the fridge with suitable foods. Some of the foods he recommends may be unfamiliar, like quinoa or the breakfast food 'Get Up & Go', and he advises dieters to track these down during the preparatory week.

In the first, 30-day phase, the aim is to switch the metabolism from storing fat to using it. *The Holford Diet* is not an 'all-you-can-eat' diet. Each food is allocated one of his GLs® figures – these are given in the book's listings, with different values allocated to different portion sizes.

Three meals and two snacks (one in the morning, one mid-afternoon) are to be eaten every day. The balance of food is critical to the diet's success: each meal should consist of 25% protein, 25% fat and 50% low-GL carbs. Clear, appetising recipes are included and there should be no reason to feel hungry.

Ground rules of the Holford Diet

- Eat up to 40 GLs® per day, choosing food containing low-GL carbs.
- Eat low-GL carbs with food rich in protein.
- Eat whole foods, high in soluble fibre.
- Eat foods high in omega-3 and omega-6 fats.
- Drink 8 glasses of water per day.
- Cut out sugar and foods containing fast-releasing carbs.
- Avoid foods high in saturated and hydrogenated fats.
- Don't eat anything to which you think you may be allergic.
- Avoid or limit alcohol.
- Avoid or limit caffeinated drinks.

Four weeks of sample menus are included. The more independent-minded dieter could use the listings to create their own meals, though Holford does advise using his menus for the first week and sticking to them as closely as you can, because they provide the correct balance of food.

Menu suggestions

Breakfast choices: porridge with berries; scrambled egg with a thin slice of rye toast; fruit yoghurt.

Lunch choices: walnut and three-bean salad with green salad; beany vegetable soup with two oat-cakes; stuffed peppers with green salad.

Dinner choices: stir-fried vegetables with tofu served with 70g brown basmati rice; tuna steak with black-eyed bean salsa and a rocket and watercress salad; chestnut and mushroom pilaf with steamed spinach and broccoli.

Snacks: apple with sunflower seeds; two oatcakes and peanut butter; cottage cheese with berries.

At the end of each week, Holford asks that you fill out a progress report, weighing and measuring yourself and recording the results. After the first 30 days he suggests

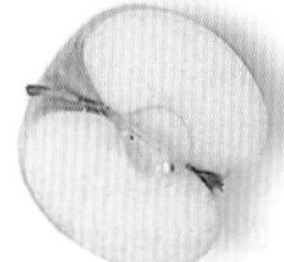

Foods to enjoy

- Fresh vegetables
- Fresh fruit
- Chicken, skinless (twice a week)
- Fish, but fatty fish like kippers, tuna and mackerel limited to 3 times per week
- Dried beans and lentils
- Rolled oats
- Rye bread, pumpernickel
- Oatcakes
- Brown rice
- Soba noodles
- Millet and quinoa

Foods to avoid

- High-fat meat – beef, pork, lamb, processed meats
- Deep-fried foods
- Cream and shop-bought ice cream
- High-fat spreads and mayo; any rich sauces
- Almost all cheese except cottage cheese, low-fat fromage frais or Quark, or half-fat cheese
- Sugar, foods with added sugar and sugar-laden sweets
- Pastries, cakes and biscuits
- White bread
- Snack foods like crisps

that if you have more weight to lose – and feel good on the diet – you should continue for up to 90 days. Once you have reached your goal you can gradually

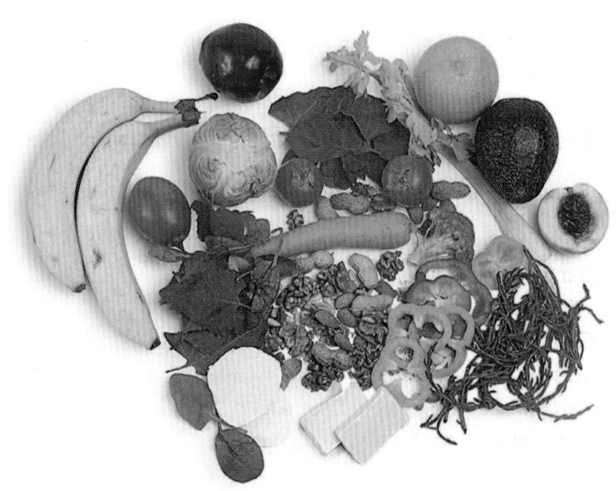

increase the number of GLs® eaten, and reduce the amount of protein from 25% to 10–15%, eating more carb-rich food. He stresses the importance of not drifting back to relying on stimulants.

Effectiveness

If you are prepared to stick to the menus and the excellent recipes provided, then this should be an effective way of losing weight. It is ideal for anyone needing a lot of support in their weight-loss efforts and, as you might expect from someone with Patrick Holford's background, there is useful psychological advice on problems like controlling compulsive eating. It is also easy for vegetarians to follow.

The diet is, however, quite demanding and may not be suitable if you require flexibility, perhaps because you are working around a family, for example. Constructing your own menus and meals is not particularly easy.

Giving up tea and coffee, not to mention chocolate and alcohol, is something that many people may find hard, and some dieters could be put off by the use of unfamiliar ingredients.

HOW TO USE THIS BOOK

The foods in this book are grouped into categories – Bakery, Biscuits, Condiments and Sauces, etc. – and listed in alphabetical order in the left-hand column of each page, together with portion sizes and cooking methods, where applicable. The emphasis is on whole foods, as these are the mainstay of GL diets.

The portion sizes given are 'average' ones that you might eat in a single serving, such as one medium apple, or 100g of chicken breast. We have also used cup measurements where they are helpful, because it's easier to visualise a cup of salad than to weigh out a specific weight of lettuce leaves, especially if you are eating in a restaurant. Note: think of a teacup-full rather than a huge mug!

The first column in the listings section gives a red, yellow or green rating to each food, according to whether it is High-GL (more than 20), Medium-GL (11 to 19) or Low-GL (10 or under). If the first column is blank, it means the food in question does not have a GL value.

For effective weight loss, concentrate on the low-GL foods; be careful with those having no value as they may be high in calories, and bear in mind the GL food pyramid on page 27. In a long-term eating plan, you just have to avoid the red-rated foods.

The second column gives the carbohydrate content of the portion in grams; the third lists its fibre content; the fourth column from the left gives the calorie count, in kilocalories, and the fifth and sixth give protein and fat counts in grams.

These portion sizes may not accord with the portion sizes your diet recommends or that you wish to eat. To find the values for a 40g piece of chicken breast, you would have to divide the figures given by 100

PASTA, RICE AND PULSES

Note that values are given for cooked products rather than raw. Pasta, rice and pulses swell up to approximately three times their weight when cooked, but food packaging often gives the values for their dry weight.

and multiply by 40. Read the weights on the packaging of any ready-prepared food as portion sizes will vary from product to product.

Values for unbranded foods have been obtained from *The Composition of Foods* (5th edition, 1991 and 6th summary edition, 2002) and *Vegetables, Herbs and Spices* (supplement, 1991), and have been reproduced by permission of Controller of Her Majesty's Stationery Office. Asda kindly supplied additional information. The publishers are grateful to all manufacturers who gave information on their products. If you cannot find a particular food here, you can obtain much fuller listings of nutrient counts in branded foods from *Collins Gem Calorie Counter* and *Collins Gem Carb Counter*.

CONVERSION CHART

Metric to imperial
100 grams (g) = 3.53 ounces (oz)
1 kilogram (kg) = 2.2 pounds (lb)
100 millilitres (ml) = 3.38 fluid ounces (fl oz)
1 litre = 1.76 pints

Imperial to metric
1 ounce (oz) = 28.35 grams (g)
1 pound (lb) = 453.60 grams (g)
1 stone (st) = 6.35 kilograms (kg)
1 fluid ounce (fl oz) = 29.57 millilitres (ml)
1 pint = 0.568 litres (l)

Abbreviations used in the listings

g	gram
kcal	kilocalorie
ml	millilitre
n/a	figures not available
—	none

The Listings

The first column in the listings section gives a red, yellow or green rating to each food, according to whether it is:

- ● High-GL (more than 20)
- ● Medium-GL (11 to 19)
- ● Low-GL (10 or under)

If the first column is blank, it means the food in question does not have a GL value.

See page 60 for further information on using the listings.

BAKERY

With bread, portion control is critical. Exceed portion size and the GL value, which is portion-dependent, can change dramatically. White bread, made with refined flour, is best avoided completely as it breaks down quickly in the digestive system; brown, 'multi-grain' and 'fortified' loaves are often made with refined flour too. Go for types with more fibre, such as stoneground wholemeal bread. Pumpernickel, sourdough and rye breads are all good choices. If comparing brands, select the one with the highest fibre count per 100g.

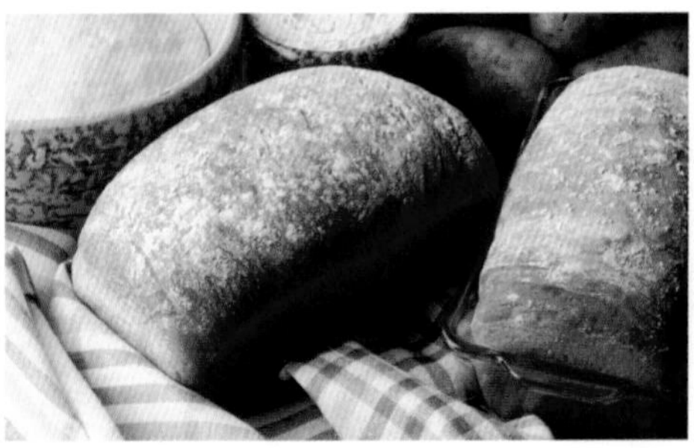

TIP: The listings give values for a slice of bread weighing about 30g, so don't kid yourself that 'one slice' means one very large or thick slice.

Food type	GL	Carb (g)	Fibre (g)	Cal (kcal)	Pro (g)	Fat (g)
Bread						
Brown, 1 slice	●	12.6	1.5	62	2.4	0.6
Brown, toasted, 1 slice	●	17.0	2.1	82	3.1	0.6
Chapattis:						
made with fat, each (50g)	○	24.2	n/a	164	4.1	6.4
made without fat, each (50g)	○	21.9	n/a	101	3.7	0.5
Ciabatta, 1 slice	●	15.5	1.0	81	3.0	1.2
Currant loaf, 1 slice	●	15.3	n/a	87	2.3	2.3
French stick, 1 slice (2cm thick)	○	18.7	1.1	88	3.0	0.6
Garlic bread, pre-packed, frozen, 1 slice	●	13.6	–	110	2.4	5.5
Granary, 1 slice	●	14.1	1.6	71	2.9	0.7
High-bran, 1 slice	○	10.2	2.4	64	4.0	0.8
Malt, 1 slice	○	19.4	1.0	88	2.3	0.7
Naan, plain, half	○	31.2	1.8	177	4.9	4.5
Oatmeal, 1 slice	●	12.4	1.1	70	2.4	1.2
Pitta bread, white, medium:	●	27.7	1.2	128	4.6	0.7
white with sesame	●	24	1.5	131	4.8	1.8
wholewheat	●	20.5	3.1	114	5.4	1.2
Pitta bread, 2 mini (10g each)	●	11.4	0.7	52	1.7	0.3
Pumpernickel, 1 slice	●	14.1	1.7	68	2.3	0.5
Rye, 1 slice	●	13.8	n/a	66	2.5	0.5
Sourdough, 1 slice	○	14.7	0.9	78	2.5	0.9
Stoneground wholemeal, 1 slice	●	11.8	2.2	65	2.9	0.7

Food type	GL	Carb (g)	Fibre (g)	Cal (kcal)	Pro (g)	Fat (g)
Wheatgerm, 1 slice	●	11.9	1.7	66	3.4	0.9
White, 1 slice	●	13.9	0.8	66	2.4	0.5
White, fried in oil/lard, 1 slice	●	14.0	0.8	149	2.4	9.7
White, toasted, 1 slice	●	17.0	0.9	81	2.9	0.6
Wholemeal, 1 slice	●	12.7	2.1	66	2.8	0.8
Rolls						
Bagels, each (70g):	●	37.2	1.5	192	7.8	1.0
onion bagels	●	37.7	1.5	192	7.8	1.1
sesame bagels	●	36.9	1.5	190	7.9	1.3
cinnamon & raisin	●	39.2	1.5	197	7.4	1.3
Baps, white, each (60g)	●	26.2	1.6	141	5.9	2.6
Brown, crusty, each (60g)	●	30.2	n/a	153	6.2	1.7
Brown, soft, each (60g)	●	26.9	2.6	142	5.9	1.9
Hamburger bun, each (60g)	●	29.2	n/a	158	5.4	3
White, crusty, each (60g)	●	32.9	1.7	157	5.5	1.3
White, soft, each (60g)	●	30.9	1.6	153	5.6	1.6
Wholemeal, each (60g)	●	27.7	3.3	147	6.3	2.0
Taco shells, each (30g)	●	18.4	n/a	152	2.1	7.8
Tortillas, each (30g):						
corn	●	18.1	n/a	103	3.0	2.1
flour	●	15.7	n/a	97	2.7	2.7

TIP: Brown bread is often made with normal white flour, but coloured with caramel or molasses. Opt for wholemeal instead.

Food type	GL	Carb (g)	Fibre (g)	Cal (kcal)	Pro (g)	Fat (g)
Tea Breads, Buns, Pastries						
Brioche, each (60g)		32.9	1.3	208	4.8	6.3
Chelsea bun, each (70g)		39.0	n/a	257	5.5	9.9
Croissant, each (70g)		30.3	2.2	261	5.8	13.8
Crumpet, each (50g)		15.9	1.5	91	3.0	0.4
Currant bun, each (70g)		36.8	2.0	196	5.6	3.9
Danish pastry, each (70g)		35.9	–	240	4.1	9.9
Doughnut, each (70g):						
jam		34.1	n/a	235	4.0	10.1
ring		33.1	–	282	4.3	15.7
Eccles cake, each (60g)		33.8	n/a	232	2.4	10.7
Fruit loaf, slice (70g)		44.9	n/a	217	4.9	3.4
Hot cross bun, each (70g)		40.9	n/a	218	5.2	4.9
Muffin, each (70g):						
English		29.5	2.3	160	7.1	1.5
blueberry		34.9	0.8	300	3	0.8
Potato scone, each (60g)		25.2	2.6	124	2.8	1.3
Raisin and cinnamon loaf, slice (70g)		35	2.2	182	4.9	2.9
Scone, each (60g):						
fruit		30.7	1.7	207	4.8	7.2

TIP: Slice bread then freeze it. You're much less likely to snack on frozen bread, but individual slices can be toasted straight from the freezer when you really need them.

Food type	GL	Carb (g)	Fibre (g)	Cal (kcal)	Pro (g)	Fat (g)
Scones *contd:*						
plain	○	32.2	n/a	218	4.3	8.9
wholemeal	○	25.9	n/a	197	5.3	8.8
Scotch pancake, each (60g)	○	29.8	0.7	158	4.0	2.7
Cakes and Cream Cakes						
Almond slice (50g bar)	●	20.6	0.8	212	6.5	12.9
Apple Danish (50g bar)	●	20.7	1.1	165	3.3	7.8
Bakewell slice (50g)	●	19.4	0.4	150	1.5	7.4
Banana cake, slice (75g)	●	41.9	0.5	260	2.4	6
Battenburg, slice (75g)	●	52.7	1.0	323	5.2	10.1
Brownies, chocolate, each (75g)	●	40.6	1.6	365	3.8	20.7
Caramel shortcake, piece (50g)	●	27.6	0.5	248	2	14.5
Carrot cake, slice (75g)	●	44.9	0.9	300	2.4	12.3
Chocolate cake, slice (75g)	●	42.3	1	268	4.3	10.5
Chocolate mini roll, each (50g)	●	27.4	0.7	222	2.2	11.1
Chocolate sandwich sponge, slice (50g)	●	24.0	0.9	192	2.0	9.8
Date and walnut loaf, slice (75g)	●	30.8	0.8	264	4.4	13.7

TIP: If you crave cake, choose a slice of fruit loaf. Many are fat-free and the dried fruit helps to reduce the GL – but don't spread it with butter.

Food type	GL	Carb (g)	Fibre (g)	Cal (kcal)	Pro (g)	Fat (g)
Chocolate éclair, each (75g)	●	19.6	n/a	297	4.2	23.0
Fancy cake, iced, each (50g)	●	34.5	–	178	1.9	4.6
Flapjack, oat, each (75g)	●	46.8	n/a	370	3.6	20.3
Fruit cake, slice (75g):						
plain	●	43.4	–	278	3.8	11.1
rich	●	44.9	n/a	257	2.9	8.5
rich, iced	●	49.4	–	263	2.7	7.4
wholemeal	●	39.3	n/a	274	4.5	12.1
Ginger cake, slice (75g)	●	46.4	0.9	295	2.6	11.0
Greek pastries (sweet), each (50g)	●	20	–	161	2.4	8.5
Lemon cake, slice (75g)	●	41.6	0.8	289	3.4	13.5
Marble cake, slice (75g)	●	41.6	0.9	278	3.9	10.5
Madeira cake, slice (75g)	●	43.8	–	283	4.1	11.3
Mince pie, each (50g)	●	30	0.8	198	1.9	7.8
Sponge cake, slice (50g):						
plain	●	26.3	n/a	234	3.2	13.6
fat-free	●	26.5	n/a	151	5	3.5
jam-filled	●	32.1	n/a	151	2.1	2.5
with butter icing	●	26.2	0.3	245	2.3	15.5
Swiss roll, original, slice (50g)	●	30.3	0.6	146	2.6	1.6
Trifle sponge, each (50g)	●	33.6	0.5	162	2.6	2.0

TIP: Be careful what you eat with your bread. Think about the fat level – and type of fat – of anything you spread on it.

BAKING PRODUCTS

GL diet books often suggest using ground almonds as a flour substitute and it is worth bearing this in mind when adapting recipes – but don't forget that ground almonds are high in calories. Whatever you use, remember to keep the fibre content high – include some stoneground wholemeal flour, for instance – to moderate the effect on the overall GL. Adding nuts and dried fruit to baking can also help.

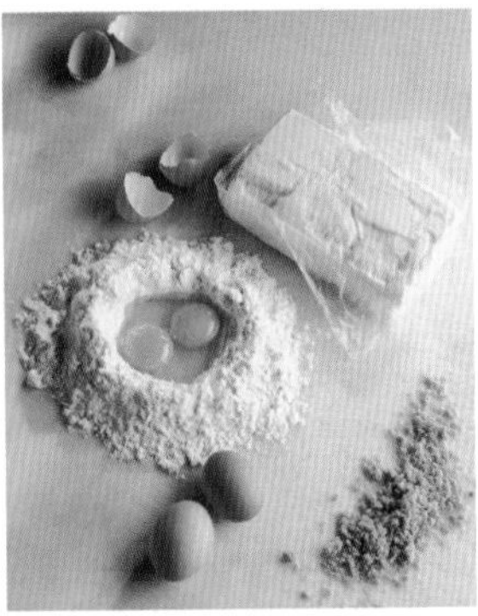

It is worth remembering that many recipes can work perfectly well with their sugar content reduced by anything up to a third. Nigel Denby's *The GL Diet* has recipes for lemon sponge cake and chocolate torte if you're a cake addict.

TIP: There are other alternatives to white flour apart from wholemeal and ground almonds. Try gram flour; it is made from chickpeas and works well in many savoury dishes.

Food type	GL	Carb (g)	Fibre (g)	Cal (kcal)	Pro (g)	Fat (g)
Baking Agents						
Baking powder, 10g (3tsp)		3.8	n/a	16	0.5	–
Cornflour, 25g		22.9	n/a	88	0.1	0.2
Flour, 100g:						
rye, whole		75.9	n/a	335	8.2	2.0
wheat, brown		68.5	n/a	324	12.6	2.0
wheat, white, breadmaking		70	3.1	337	11.0	1.4
wheat, white, plain		71	3.1	336	10.0	1.3
wheat, white, self-raising		72	2.0	343	11.0	1.2
wheat, wholemeal		58.0	9	308	14.0	2.2
Ground rice, 100g		86.8	0.5	361	6.5	1
Pastry, 50g:						
filo, uncooked		31	1	156	4.5	1.5
flaky, cooked		23	n/a	282	2.8	20.5
puff, uncooked		15	0.8	210	2.5	15.5
shortcrust, cooked		27.2	n/a	262	3.3	16.3
shortcrust, mix		30.4	1.2	234	3.7	11.6
wholemeal, cooked		22.3	n/a	251	4.5	16.6
Sugar, caster, 50g		50	–	200	–	–
Yeast, bakers'						
compressed, 25g		0.3	n/a	13	2.9	0.1
dried, 15g		0.5	n/a	25	5.3	0.2

TIP: Traditional milling processes preserve more nutrients and fibre than modern rolling mills, so opt for old-fashioned stoneground flours.

Food type	GL	Carb (g)	Fibre (g)	Cal (kcal)	Pro (g)	Fat (g)
Fats						
Butter, 25g		Tr	n/a	225	Tr	25
Cooking fat, 25g		–	–	225	–	25
Lard, 1tbsp		–	n/a	134	Tr	14.9
Margarine, hard (over 80% animal/vegetable fat), 25g		0.3	n/a	180	0.1	19.8
Margarine, soft (over 80% polyunsaturated fat), 25g		0.1	n/a	187	Tr	20.7
Suet, shredded, 1 tbsp		1.8	n/a	124	Tr	13
Mixes						
Batter mix, 100g		77.2	3.7	338	9.3	1.2
Cheesecake mix, 100g:						
strawberry		31.5	n/a	258	3	12
toffee		37.5	n/a	342	3.2	19.3
Crumble mix, 100g		67.6	1.5	422	5.5	16.3
Egg custard mix, no bake, 100g		14.1	0.5	96	4.4	2.4
Madeira cake mix, 100g		56	n/a	339	4.9	12.4
Pancake mix, 100g		65.9	2.3	322	13.4	2.5
Victoria sponge mix, 100g		52	n/a	367	6	15

TIP: Try using fructose in baking rather than ordinary sugar. It has a lower GL and is also sweeter, so you will need less of it. Note that it cooks at lower temperatures – most packs provide accurate guidance.

Food type	GL	Carb (g)	Fibre (g)	Cal (kcal)	Pro (g)	Fat (g)
Sundries						
Almonds, flaked/ground, 25g		1.8	1.8	158	6.3	14
Cherries, *glacé*, 25g		16.6	n/a	63	0.1	–
Cherry pie filling, 100g		21.5	n/a	82	0.4	Tr
Currants, dried, 25g		17	n/a	67	0.6	0.1
Ginger, glacé, 25g		18.6	n/a	76	0.1	0.2
Lemon juice, 50ml		0.8	n/a	4	0.2	Tr
Marzipan, 50g		33.8	–	195	2.7	6.4
Mincemeat (sweet), 50g		31.1	n/a	137	0.3	2.2
Mixed peel, 25g		14.8	n/a	58	0.1	0.2
Raisins, seedless, 25g		17.3	0.5	72	0.5	0.1
Royal icing, 50g		48.8	–	195	0.7	–
Sultanas, 25g		17.4	0.5	69	0.7	0.1

TIP: Avoid pre-prepared baking mixes as most are very high in calories and high GL. Making your own mixtures doesn't take long, and you control the ingredients.

BEANS, PULSES AND CEREALS

Pulses and beans are almost all low GL, and they are an excellent source of other nutrients beside carbs: protein, fibre, minerals and vitamins. Adding them to casseroles, salads and soups slows down the digestive process. Dried beans are cheaper, but most need soaking overnight, draining and boiling in fresh water for about 10 minutes before being simmered at a lower temperature until tender. Once cooked, they keep for a few days in the fridge and can also be frozen. Tinned beans are an excellent standby and generally only need draining and rinsing before use.

TIP: Make a bean salad with dried black-eye beans, haricot beans and butter beans. Soak them overnight, then cook them with a chopped onion and a bay leaf; when they are soft, drain them and allow to cool. Before they are completely cold, dress them with lemon juice and olive oil, some chopped parsley, salt and black pepper; add chopped black olives and mix thoroughly. Serve decorated with slices of hard-boiled egg and some whole olives.

Food type	GL	Carb (g)	Fibre (g)	Cal (kcal)	Pro (g)	Fat (g)
Beans and Pulses						
Aduki beans, 115g	●	25.9	n/a	141	10.7	0.2
Baked beans, small can (200g):						
in tomato sauce	●	30.6	n/a	168	10.4	1.2
tomato sauce, no added sugar	●	22.6	7.4	132	9.4	0.4
Baked beans with pork sausages, small can (200g)	●	22.0	6.0	194	11.2	6.8
Baked beans with vegetable sausages, small can (200g)	●	24.4	5.8	210	12.0	7.2
Blackeyed beans, 115g	●	22.9	n/a	133	10.1	0.8
Borlotti beans, half can (100g)	●	20.5	5.5	121	8.7	0.5
Broad beans, small can (200g)	●	22	10	164	16	1.4
Butter beans:						
small can (200g)	●	27.8	9.6	166	12.0	0.8
dried, boiled (115g)	●	21.2	6	118	8.2	0.7
Cannellini beans, *small can* (200g)	●	28	12	174	14	0.6
Chick peas:						
small can (200g)	●	32.2	n/a	230	14.4	5.8
dried, boiled (115g)	●	20.9	n/a	139	9.7	2.4

TIP: A fresh lentil salad, with a little raw red onion and fresh herbs mixed with the cooked lentils, is delicious. Mix an oil and vinegar dressing at least 30 minutes before serving so the flavours can develop.

Food type	GL	Carb (g)	Fibre (g)	Cal (kcal)	Pro (g)	Fat (g)
Chilli beans, small can (200g)	●	28	7.4	160	9.6	1
Flageolet beans, half can (100g)	●	22.4	2.4	132	9.0	0.7
Haricot beans, 115g						
dried, boiled	●	19.8	7	109	7.6	0.6
Hummus, 2 tbsp	●	3.3	n/a	53	2.2	3.6
Lentils, 115g:						
green/brown, boiled	●	19.4	n/a	121	10.1	0.8
red, split, boiled	●	20.1	n/a	115	8.7	0.5
Marrow fat peas:						
small can (200g)	●	28	9.6	168	12	0.8
quick-soak, 115g	●	48.2	16.1	334	29.1	2.8
Mung beans, 115g						
boiled	●	17.6	n/a	105	8.7	0.5
Pinto beans:						
boiled, 115g	●	27.5	–	158	10.2	0.8
refried, 2 tbsp	●	4.6	–	32	1.9	0.3
Red kidney beans:						
small can (200g)	●	27	12.8	182	16.2	1.0
boiled, 115g	●	20	n/a	118	9.7	0.6
Soya beans, 115g						
dried, boiled	●	5.9	n/a	162	16.1	8.4

TIP: Try using soaked and cooked dried beans, or tinned ones, to replace some of the meat in family favourites like shepherd's pie, stews, moussaka or lasagne.

Food type	GL	Carb (g)	Fibre (g)	Cal (kcal)	Pro (g)	Fat (g)
Split peas, 115g, *boiled*	●	26.1	3.1	1454	9.5	1
Tofu (soya bean curd), 2 tbsp:						
steamed	●	0.9	–	94	10.4	5.4
fried	●	2.6	–	337	30.3	22.9
Cereals						
Barley, pearl, 100g	●	83.6	7.3	360	7.9	1.7
Bran, 100g:						
wheat, dry	●	26.8	n/a	206	14.1	5.5
Bulgur wheat, dry, 100g	●	74	3.1	357	12	1.4
Couscous, dry, 100g	●	72.5	2	355	13.5	1.9
Cracked wheat, 100g	●	74	3.1	357	12	1.4
Polenta, ready-made, 100g	●	15.7	n/a	72	1.6	0.3
Wheatgerm, 100g	●	44.7	n/a	357	26.7	9.2
Fresh beans & peas:						
see Vegetables						
For more soya products:						
see Vegetarian						

TIP: You can keep dried beans for years but they get drier and harder as they get older, becoming resistant to soaking and cooking. It's best to buy small quantities at a time, and don't buy any packs that look dusty. Keep beans in airtight containers.

BISCUITS, CRACKERS AND CRISPBREADS

Some biscuits may have a low GL, but think about the calorie content – and about whether you can stop at one – before deciding to eat them. If you do, go for those with ingredients that boost the fibre count, like dried fruit or wholegrains. Read labels carefully, as trans fats seem to be ubiquitous in shop-bought biscuits these days. Oatcakes can be very useful on a GL diet. Rough oatcakes have a lower fat content than fine ones, and bran oatcakes have double the fibre of rough ones. They are delicious spread thinly with hummus.

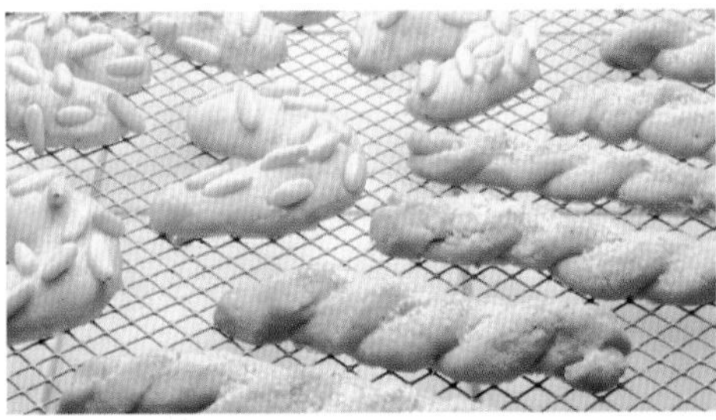

TIP: Trans fats, sometimes called hydrogenates or hydrogenated fats on labels, started life as polyunsaturated fats but processing at high temperatures changed their chemical structure. They are associated with an increased risk of heart disease and certain cancers.

Food type	GL	Carb (g)	Fibre (g)	Cal (kcal)	Pro (g)	Fat (g)
Sweet Biscuits						
Bourbon creams, each	●	7	n/a	47	n/a	1.9
Caramel wafers, each	●	6.7	n/a	45	0.5	2
Chocolate chip cookies, each	●	5.7	n/a	43	0.6	2
Chocolate cream wafers, each	●	3.2	n/a	26	0.3	1.4
Chocolate fingers, each:						
milk & plain chocolate	●	6.3	n/a	52	0.7	2.7
white chocolate	●	6.1	n/a	53	0.6	3
Shortcake cream sandwich						
fruit	●	9.2	0.3	75	0.9	3.8
milk chocolate	●	9.4	0.3	77	0.9	3.9
mint	●	9.4	0.3	78	0.8	4
orange	●	9.3	0.3	78	0.8	4.1
Custard creams, each	●	6.9	0.2	51	0.6	2.3
Digestive biscuits, each:						
uncoated	●	8.6	–	58	0.8	2.5
chocolate (milk & plain)	●	10	–	74	1	3.6
Fig rolls each	●	6.8	0.5	36	0.4	0.8
Garibaldi (plain), each	●	7.1	0.3	40	0.5	1.0
Gingernuts, each	●	8	–	44	0.6	1.3
Gipsy creams, each	●	9.9	0.4	77	0.7	3.8
Jaffa cakes, each	●	7.0	0.2	37	0.5	0.8
Lemon puff, each	●	6.2	0.2	52	0.7	2.7
Nice biscuits, each	●	6.9	0.2	49	0.7	2.1
Oat & raisin biscuits, each	●	6.3	0.4	47	0.8	2.1

Food type	GL	Carb (g)	Fibre (g)	Cal (kcal)	Pro (g)	Fat (g)
Rich tea biscuits, each		7.2	0.3	46	0.7	1.6
Shortbread fingers, each		12.8	0.4	100	1.2	5.2
Shortcake biscuits, each		6.5	n/a	49	0.6	2.3
Stem ginger cookies, diet, each		6.5	0.1	40	0.5	1.3
Viennese whirls, each		2.3	0.1	21	0.2	1.3
Wafer biscuits, cream-filled, each		4.6	–	37	0.3	2.1
Crackers and Crispbreads						
Bran crackers, 4		12.6	0.6	91	1.9	3.6
Cheese crackers , 4		8.3	0.4	81	1.5	4.7
Cornish wafers, each		5.4	0.2	53	0.8	3.1
Crackerbread, each:						
original		7.6	0.3	38	1	0.3
cheese-flavoured		7.5	0.3	38	1.3	0.3
high-fibre		6.2	1.6	32	1.3	0.3
Crackers, salted, 5:						
cheese		8.4	0.3	74	1.6	3.8
original		8.3	0.3	76	1	4.3
Cream crackers, each		5.7	0.3	36	0.8	1.1
Matzo crackers, each		8.5	0.3	37	1	0.2
Oatcakes, each:						
cheese		5.4	0.6	47	1.3	2.5

TIP: Biscuits which contain dried fruit may have a lower GL, but don't eat more than one a day if you're serious about losing weight.

Food type	**GL**	**Carb (g)**	**Fibre (g)**	**Cal (kcal)**	**Pro (g)**	**Fat (g)**
Oatcakes, *contd*:						
fine	●	6.3	0.9	46	1	2.2
organic	●	7.1	0.9	42	0.9	1.6
rough	●	6.4	0.8	43	1.2	1.8
traditional	●	5.8	0.8	43	1.1	1.7
Rye crispbread, each:						
dark rye	○	6.5	1.8	31	0.9	0.1
multigrain	○	5.7	1.7	33	1.1	0.6
original	○	6.7	1.7	33	1.1	0.1
sesame	○	6	1.6	34	0.9	0.6
Water biscuits, 3:						
high bake	○	7.6	0.3	41	1	0.7
regular (table)	○	7.5	0.4	41	1	0.8
Wholemeal crackers, 4	○	10.8	0.7	62	1.5	1.7
See also *Snacks and dips*						

TIP: Oatcakes are a good choice, but try to select ones which don't contain palm oil, a saturated fat. Those made with olive oil are better for you.

BREAKFAST CEREALS AND CEREAL BARS

On any GL diet, and on most others, breakfast is an essential meal; studies have shown that people who skip it are more likely to be overweight, partly because slow-release carbs help you to avoid the mid-morning munchies. Porridge is often recommended, but don't buy quick-cook or instant oats. It can be enlivened with fresh or frozen fruit, dried apricots or low-fat yoghurt. With cold cereals, choose those containing bran or oats but without sugar, or try making your own muesli. Avoid anything slathered in sugar or chocolate, and approach cereal bars with caution.

TIP: Add a few finely chopped dried apricots just before your porridge is ready, and serve it with a dollop of no-fat Greek yoghurt.

Food type	GL	Carb (g)	Fibre (g)	Cal (kcal)	Pro (g)	Fat (g)
Breakfast Cereals						
Bran flakes, 30g	●	19.8	4.5	97	3	0.6
Cheerios, 40g:	●	30.1	2.6	148	3.2	1.6
honey-nut	●	31.3	2.1	150	2.8	1.5
Cornflakes, 30g:	●	23.4	0.9	112	2.1	0.3
Crunchy nut	●	24.9	0.8	118	1.8	1.2
Sugar coated	●	26.1	0.6	111	1.4	0.2
Chocolate sugar coated	●	24.0	1.1	118	1.5	1.8
Fruit 'n' Fibre, 30g	●	20.4	2.7	107	2.4	1.8
Grape Nuts, 40g	●	29	3.4	138	4.2	0.8
High Fibre Bran, 40g	●	18.4	10.8	112	5.6	1.8
Low fat flakes, 30g:	●	22.5	0.8	112	4.8	0.3
with red berries	●	22.8	0.9	111	4.2	0.3
Malted Wheats, 30g	●	21.9	2.8	108	3.2	0.8
Multi-grain cereal, 30g	●	24	1.5	113	2.4	0.8
Oat Bran Flakes, 30g	●	20.1	0.6	99	3	0.6
Oat Krunchies, 30g	●	18.9	3.3	108	3.2	2.1
Puffed Rice, 30g:	●	26.1	0.3	114	1.8	0.3
chocolate	●	25.2	0.6	115	1.5	0.9
sugar coated	●	27	0.3	115	1.4	0.2
Puffed Wheat, 30g	●	18.7	1.7	98	4.6	0.4

TIP: Put porridge on to cook while you get on with your morning tasks, but remember to stir it occasionally. You will learn to judge how much you can do – perhaps washing and dressing – before it is ready.

Food type	GL	Carb (g)	Fibre (g)	Cal (kcal)	Pro (g)	Fat (g)
Shredded wheat bisks, 30g:		20.3	3.5	102	3.5	0.8
bitesize		21.0	3.6	105	3.5	0.8
sugar coated		21.6	2.7	105	3	0.6
fruit-filled		20.6	2.7	106	2.5	1.5
honey nut		20.6	2.8	113	3.4	2
Sultana Bran, 30g		20.1	0.4	95	2.4	0.6
Wheat bisks , 30g		20.4	3.0	101	3.5	0.6
Hot Cereals						
Instant Porridge						
baked apple		71	5.5	374	8	6
berry burst		71	5.5	374	8	6
golden syrup		71	6	372	7.5	6
Oatbran, 100g		49.7	15.2	345	14.8	9.7
Oatmeal, medium or fine, 100g		60.4	8.5	359	11	8.1
Oats, 100g:						
instant		60.4	8.5	359	11	8.1
jumbo		60.4	8.5	359	11	8.1
organic		61.5	8.0	363	12.5	7.4
rolled		62	7	368	11	8

TIP: A couple of apples and a handful of nuts are a better choice than a cereal bar for the GL dieter. Most cereal bars on the market are sugar-coated and often have extra sweeteners on top. Muesli bars with dried fruits and seeds may look healthy but can also be loaded with sugar.

Food type	GL	Carb (g)	Fibre (g)	Cal (kcal)	Pro (g)	Fat (g)
Porridge (cooked), 100g:						
made with water	●	8.1	n/a	46	1.4	1.1
made with whole milk	●	12.6	n/a	113	4.8	5.1
Muesli						
Crunchy Oat Cereal, 50g:						
maple & pecan	○	30.0	3.3	224	5	9.4
raisin & almond	○	33	2.8	211	3.5	7.2
sultana & apple	○	29.6	6.2	189	3.8	6.1
Muesli, 50g:	●	33	3.8	182	5	3.4
apricot	●	29.5	2.8	142	3.9	1.8
deluxe	●	28.1	5.8	172	5.4	5
high fibre	●	35.4	3	158	5.2	3
natural	●	31.5	4.3	173	4.8	3.1
organic	●	29.8	4.5	177	4.5	4.4
swiss-style	●	36.1	n/a	182	4.9	3
swiss-style, organic	●	31.5	3.7	180	4.9	3.8
with no added sugar	●	33.6	n/a	183	5.3	3.9

TIP: Make your own muesli. Mix 450g porridge oats with 50g oat bran, 2 tablespoons each of sunflower seeds, pumpkin seeds and chopped nuts, plus a tablespoon of linseed. For toasted muesli, put this mixture in an ovenproof dish and bake at 200°C/gas mark 6 for about 15 minutes until it looks golden; stir once during this time. Once it has cooled add 50g chopped dried apricots. Mix well and store in an airtight jar.

Food type	GL	Carb (g)	Fibre (g)	Cal (kcal)	Pro (g)	Fat (g)
Cereal Bars						
Apple & blackberry, 30g	●	20.8	1.5	117	1.6	3.1
Banana, 30g	●	27.6	2	152	2.3	2
Cornflakes & milk bar, 30g	○	19.8	0.6	132	2.7	4.8
Fruit & Nut Break, 30g	○	23.7	2	170	3.0	7.0
Fruit and oats crisp, 30g:						
Apricot	●	21.3	2.1	122	1.7	3.3
Raisin & Hazelnut	●	20.4	1.3	142	2.1	5.8
Low fat flakes & milk bar, 30g	○	20.7	0.4	135	2.1	4.8
Muesli bar, 30g	○	30.6	2	178	2.7	5
Multi-grain bar, 30g:						
Apple	○	19.8	1.1	106	1.2	2.7
Cappuccino	○	19.8	0.7	111	1.4	3
Cherry	○	20.1	1.2	104	1.2	2.4
Chocolate	○	19.8	1.2	110	1.4	3.0
Orange	○	19.5	1.2	105	1.2	2.7
Strawberry	○	20.1	1.1	107	1.2	2.7
Oat and wheat bar, 30g:	○	22.5	0.6	117	2.1	2.1
Chocolate chip	○	17.7	0.5	147	2.1	7.2
Roasted nut	○	16.4	0.4	151	2.7	8

TIP: Most breakfast cereals have a lot of added sugar, even some of the 'healthy' or 'vitamin-enriched' ones. Go for those based on bran or oats, but still check labels carefully. Top them with skimmed milk, or low-fat, unsweetened soya milk with added calcium.

Food type	GL	Carb (g)	Fibre (g)	Cal (kcal)	Pro (g)	Fat (g)
Puffed rice & milk bar, 30g	●	20.4	0.1	124	2.1	3.9
Strawberry & yoghurt, 30g	●	21.0	1.1	119	1.7	3.1
Sugar coated flakes & milk bar, 30g	●	20.7	0.5	114	2.4	4.5

TIP: Liven up your breakfast cereal with fresh fruit – grated apple is refreshing – or a little dried fruit. Choose something a bit unusual like dried cranberries or strawberries, but use in moderation.

CONDIMENTS, SAUCES AND GRAVY

Shop-bought cooking sauces are best avoided completely on a GL diet because they are often high in sugar and/or flour. Commercial chutneys can also be problematic. It is, however, fine to use a couple of teaspoons of the low-GL table sauces listed in this section. Stick to portion sizes carefully as overdoing it would mean a considerable extra batch of calories as well as blowing the GL of your meal. Some are better than others; mustard can be useful for cooking as well as accompanying meat – add a little Dijon mustard to dips, yoghurt dressings, soups and casseroles for a depth of flavour.

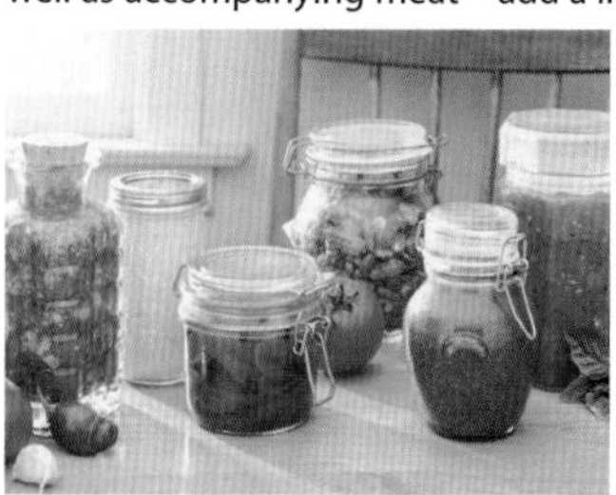

TIP: To make a quick salad dressing put oil and lemon juice in a screw-top jar, add a little black pepper and a small amount of Dijon mustard. Close the jar firmly and shake it to mix the vinaigrette. It can be kept in the fridge; remove it about 30 minutes before use, and shake it thoroughly before drizzling over your salad.

Food type	GL	Carb (g)	Fibre (g)	Cal (kcal)	Pro (g)	Fat (g)
Table Sauces						
Apple sauce, 1 tbsp	●	4	0.2	16	–	Tr
Barbecue sauce, 1 tbsp	●	4.1	0.1	18	0.1	–
Beetroot in redcurrant jelly 1 tbsp	●	6.1	n/a	25	0.1	Tr
Brown fruity sauce, 1 tbsp	●	3.6	0.2	17	0.1	–
Brown sauce, 1 tbsp	●	3.4	n/a	15	0.2	–
Burger sauce, 1 tbsp	●	1.8	Tr	36	0.2	3.1
Chilli sauce, 1 tsp	●	1.7	–	7	0.1	Tr
Cranberry jelly, 1 tbsp	●	10	–	40	Tr	Tr
Cranberry sauce, 1 tbsp	●	6.8	n/a	27	–	–
Garlic sauce, 1 tsp	●	0.9	n/a	17	0.1	1.5
Ginger sauce, 1 tsp	●	1.4	–	6	–	–
Horseradish, creamed, 2 tsp	●	2	0.2	18	0.2	1
Horseradish relish, 2 tsp	●	1	0.3	11	0.2	0.6
Horseradish sauce, 2 tsp	●	1.8	n/a	15	0.2	0.8
Mint jelly, 1 tbsp	●	10	n/a	40	Tr	–
Mint sauce, 1 tbsp	●	1.9	n/a	9	0.2	–
Mushroom ketchup, 1 tbsp	●	0.8	Tr	4	0.1	–
Redcurrant jelly, 1 tbsp	●	9.8	n/a	39	–	–
Soy sauce, 2 tsp	●	0.8	n/a	4	0.3	Tr

TIP: Make your own apple sauce by blending some unsweetened stewed apples until they are still slightly rough in texture. The better the quality of the apples you use, the better your sauce will be.

Food type	GL	Carb (g)	Fibre (g)	Cal (kcal)	Pro (g)	Fat (g)
Tabasco, 1 tsp		–	–	–	–	–
Tartare sauce, 1 tbsp	●	1.3	n/a	77	0.1	7.9
Tomato ketchup, 1 tbsp	●	4.7	n/a	19	0.3	–
Wild rowan jelly, 2 tsp	●	6.5	n/a	27	–	–
Worcestershire sauce, 1 tsp	●	1.0	–	4	–	–
Mustards						
Dijon mustard, 1 tsp	●	0.1	0.1	5	0.3	0.4
English mustard, 1 tsp	●	0.9	0.1	9	0.3	0.4
French mustard, 1 tsp	●	0.6	–	7	0.3	0.3
Honey mustard, 1 tsp	●	1.2	0.3	9	0.3	0.2
Horseradish mustard, 1 tsp	●	1.2	0.2	8	0.3	0.2
Peppercorn mustard, 1 tsp	●	0.8	0.3	7	0.4	0.3
Wholegrain mustard, 1tsp:	●	0.5	0.2	8	0.5	0.5
hot, 1 tsp	●	0.6	0.4	7	0.4	0.2
Pickles and Chutneys						
Apple chutney, 1 tbsp	●	7.3	n/a	28	0.1	–
Barbecue relish, 1 tbsp	●	3.1	n/a	14	0.3	–
Chunky fruit chutney, 1 tbsp:	●	3.9	n/a	16	0.1	–
small chunk	●	–	0.2	21	0.1	–

TIP: A simple cranberry sauce can liven up fish as well as poultry. Make your own by cooking fresh cranberries with a little water over a moderate heat until they pop, then stir in a little sugar and serve warm or cold.

Food type	GL	Carb (g)	Fibre (g)	Cal (kcal)	Pro (g)	Fat (g)
Chunky fruit chutney, *contd*:						
spicy		5.1	0.2	21	0.1	–
Lime pickle, 1 tbsp		0.6	0.1	29	0.3	2.8
Mango chutney, 1 tbsp		7.5	0.2	31	0.1	–
Mango with ginger chutney						
1 tbsp		6.9	0.1	28	0.1	–
Mediterranean chutney, 1 tbsp		3.9	0.2	17.9	0.3	0.1
Mustard pickle, mild, 1 tbsp		3.8	0.1	19	0.3	0.2
Piccalilli, 1 tbsp		3.2	0.1	16	0.2	0.1
Ploughman's pickle, 1 tbsp		4	0.1	17	0.1	–
Sandwich pickle, tangy, 1 tbsp		4.7	0.1	20	0.1	–
Sauerkraut, 2 tbsp		0.4	n/a	3	0.4	Tr
Spiced fruit chutney, 1 tbsp		5.1	n/a	21	0.1	–
Spreadable chutney, 1 tbsp		8.8	0.2	36	–	–
Sweet chilli dipping sauce,						
1 tbsp		7.8	0.1	33	0.1	–
Sweet pickle, 1 tbsp		5.4	n/a	21	0.1	–
Tomato chutney, 1 tbsp		4.6	n/a	19	0.2	–
Tomato pickle, tangy, 1 tbsp		5.2	0.4	25	0.5	–
Tomato with red pepper						
chutney, 1 tbsp		5.7	0.2	25	0.3	

TIP: Use a tomato salsa – a mixture of finely chopped tomatoes, coriander, red onions, lime juice and an optional chopped chilli – instead of tomato ketchup.

Food type	GL	Carb (g)	Fibre (g)	Cal (kcal)	Pro (g)	Fat (g)
Salad Dressings						
Balsamic dressing, 2 tbsp	●	2.2	–	92	0.1	9.1
Blue cheese dressing, 2 tbsp	●	2.6	n/a	137	0.6	13.9
Blue cheese-flavoured low-fat dressing, 2 tbsp	●	1.8	–	18	0.5	1
Creamy Caesar dressing, 2 tbsp	●	2.4	–	101	0.9	9.6
Caesar-style low-fat dressing, 2 tbsp	●	4.4	0.1	24	1	0.3
Creamy low-fat salad dressing, 2 tbsp	●	4.5	n/a	37	0.2	2
French dressing, 2 tbsp	●	1.4	–	139	–	14.9
Italian dressing, 2 tbsp	●	1.7	0.1	36	–	3.1
fat free	●	2	0.2	10	–	Tr
Mayonnaise, 1 tbsp	●	0.3	–	109	0.2	11.9
light, reduced calorie, 1 tbsp	●	2.5	0.2	96	0.3	9.5
Salad cream, 1 tbsp	●	2.5	–	52	0.2	4.7
light, 1 tbsp	●	2	Tr	36	0.3	3
Seafood sauce, 1 tbsp	●	1.5	0.1	80	0.3	8.1
Thousand Island, 1 tbsp	●	2.9	0.1	55	0.1	4.7
fat free, 1 tbsp	●	3	0.4	13	0.1	–
Vinaigrette, 2 tbsp	●	1.4	–	139	–	14.8

TIP: Tabasco sauce is a good way to perk up soups, casseroles, even salad dressings. It is made from the powerful tabasco chilli pepper, so go easy; you only need a few drops to make a difference.

Food type	GL	Carb (g)	Fibre (g)	Cal (kcal)	Pro (g)	Fat (g)
Vinegars						
Balsamic vinegar, 1 tbsp	●	3.2	–	15	Tr	–
Cider vinegar, 1 tbsp	●	0.2	–	3	–	–
Red wine vinegar, 1 tbsp	●	0.1	–	4	–	–
Sherry vinegar, 1 tbsp	●	0.3	–	4	0.1	–
White wine vinegar, 1 tbsp	●	0.1	–	3	–	–
Cooking Sauces						
Bread sauce, 100ml:						
made with semi-skimmed milk	●	15.3	n/a	97	4.2	2.5
made with whole milk	●	15.2	n/a	110	4.1	4
Cheese sauce, 100ml:						
made with semi-skimmed milk	●	8.8	n/a	181	8.2	12.8
made with whole milk	●	8.7	n/a	198	8.1	14.8
Curry sauce, canned, 100ml	●	7.1	n/a	78	1.5	5
Onion sauce, 100ml:						
made with semi-skimmed milk	●	8.2	n/a	88	3	5.1
made with whole milk	●	8.1	n/a	101	2.9	6.6
Pesto:						
fresh, homemade 100ml	●	6	1.4	45	2.2	1.3
green pesto, jar, 100ml	●	0.8	1.4	374	5	39

TIP: To lower the calorie count of low-fat mayonnaise further, mix it with the same quantity of no-fat Greek yoghurt. Add some chopped chives or fresh herbs, such as coriander, to make it special.

Food type	GL	Carb (g)	Fibre (g)	Cal (kcal)	Pro (g)	Fat (g)
Pesto *contd:*						
red pesto, jar, 100ml		3.1	0.4	358	4.1	36.6
Tomato & basil, fresh, 100ml		8.8	1.3	51	1.8	0.9
White sauce, 100ml:						
made with semi-skimmed milk		10.7	n/a	130	4.4	8
made with whole milk		10.6	n/a	151	4.2	10.3
For more pasta sauces, *see under: Pasta and Pizza*						
Stock Cubes						
Beef, each		2.3	Tr	32	0.9	2.3
Chicken, each		2.3	Tr	32	0.9	1.8
Fish, each		0.5	Tr	32	1.8	2.3
Garlic herb & spice, each		5.3	0.4	33	1.5	0.6
Ham , each		1.8	Tr	32	1.4	1.8
Lamb, each		0.5	Tr	32	1.4	2.3
Rice saffron, each		1.4	0.4	32	1.6	2.2
Pork, each		1.4	Tr	32	1.4	2.3
Vegetable, each		1.4	Tr	45	1.4	4.1
Yeast extract, each		2.8	n/a	27	2.7	0.5

TIP: Try using low-fat natural yoghurt as a salad dressing rather than oil and vinegar. Add chopped cucumber to make tzatziki, or stir in some Dijon mustard for a spicier taste.

Food type	GL	Carb (g)	Fibre (g)	Cal (kcal)	Pro (g)	Fat (g)
Gravy Granules						
Gravy powder, 5g	●	3.1	–	13	0.1	–
Gravy instant granules, 5g	●	2.9	0.1	19	0.1	0.8
Swiss Vegetable Bouillon powder, 4g	●	0.7	n/a	4	0.3	–
Vegetable gravy granules, 5g	●	3	0.2	15	0.4	0.2

TIP: When buying soy sauce, be aware that many popular varieties have added caramel: check for sugars on the label and buy one that is naturally fermented instead. Shoyu is the term for lighter soy sauce; tamari is the darker, stronger type.

DAIRY

Dairy foods have no GL unless they contain some added carbs, like apricots in cheese. However, if you want to lose weight you need to remember that dairy products can be very high in calories and that cream, butter and cheese are all generally high in saturated fat. Choose low- or no-fat versions and change to skimmed milk. If you find skimmed milk unpalatable initially, then change gradually, going to semi-skimmed first (but always use skimmed in cooking). Watch the quantities of cheese you use; swap to lower-fat types like Edam, mozzarella and feta.

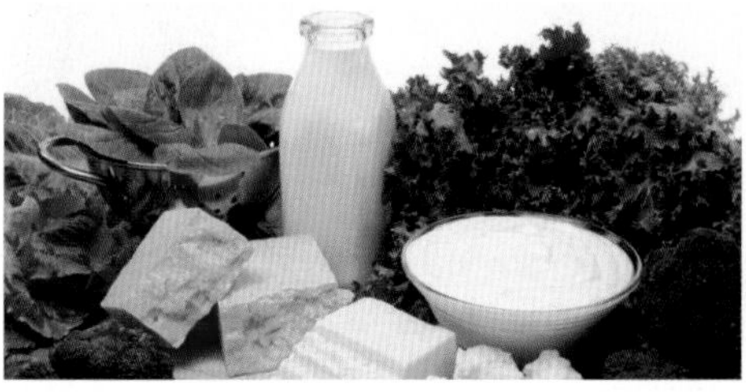

TIP: Watch out for trans fats (aka hydrogenates or hydrogenated fats) in margarines and spreads. Try olive oil-based spreads, or just drizzle a little olive oil on your bread. Really tasty bread may not need anything on it, especially if it's accompanying soup.

Food type	GL	Carb (g)	Fibre (g)	Cal (kcal)	Pro (g)	Fat (g)
Milk and Cream						
Buttermilk, 250ml		20.3	n/a	138	14.3	Tr
Cream:						
extra thick, 2 tbsp		1.1	–	70	0.8	6.9
fresh, clotted, 2 tbsp		0.7	n/a	176	0.5	19.1
fresh, double, 2 tbsp		0.5	–	149	0.5	16.1
fresh, single, 2 tbsp		0.7	–	58	1	5.7
fresh, soured, 2 tbsp		0.9	n/a	62	0.9	6.0
fresh, whipping, 2 tbsp		0.8	–	114	0.6	12
sterilised, canned, 2 tbsp		1.2	n/a	76	0.8	7.6
UHT, aerosol spray, 2 tbsp		2.5	–	86	0.6	8.3
UHT, double, vegetarian, 2 tbsp		1.2	0.2	92	0.8	9.3
UHT, single, vegetarian, 2 tbsp		1.4	0.1	44	0.9	3.9
Crème fraiche:						
full fat, 2 tbsp		0.7	–	113	0.7	12
half fat, 2 tbsp		1.3	–	49	0.8	4.5
Milk, fresh:						
cows', whole, 250ml		11.3	n/a	165	8.3	9.8
cows', semi-skimmed, 250ml		11.8	–	115	8.5	4.3
cows', skimmed, 250ml		11	–	80	8.5	0.5
cows', Channel Island, 250ml		12	n/a	195	9	12.8

TIP: Use low- or no-fat dairy products when possible but check the ingredient lists. Some low-fat products, particularly fruit yoghurts, may be high in sugar.

Food type	GL	Carb (g)	Fibre (g)	Cal (kcal)	Pro (g)	Fat (g)
Milk, *contd:*						
goats', pasteurised, 250ml	●	11	–	155	7.8	9.3
sheep's, 250ml	●	12.8	–	233	13.5	14.5
Milk, evaporated:						
original, 100ml	●	11.5	–	160	8.2	9
light, 100ml	●	10.5	–	110	7.5	4
Milk, dried, skimmed, 250ml	●	75.5	n/a	515	51.5	0.8
Milk, condensed:						
whole milk, sweetened, 100ml	●	55.5	n/a	333	8.5	10.1
skimmed milk, sweetened, 100ml	●	60	n/a	267	10	0.2
Soya milk:						
unsweetened, 250ml	●	1.3	1.3	65	6	4
sweetened, 250ml	●	6.3	Tr	108	7.8	6
Rice drink:						
calcium enriched, 250ml	●	24	–	125	0.3	3
vanilla, organic, 250ml	●	23.8	–	123	0.3	3
Yoghurt and Fromage Frais						
Diet yoghurts, 125g:						
banana	●	10.9	n/a	66	5.5	0.1
cherry	●	9.9	n/a	63	5.5	0.1
vanilla	●	10.4	n/a	66	5.8	0.1

TIP: Low-fat crème fraîche is stable when heated, unlike some dairy products, and is therefore great to use in cooking – in sauces, for example.

Food type	GL	Carb (g)	Fibre (g)	Cal (kcal)	Pro (g)	Fat (g)
Fromage frais, 1 pot (50g):						
fruit	●	7	Tr	62	2.7	2.8
plain	●	2.2	–	57	3.1	4
virtually fat free, fruit	●	2.8	0.4	25	3.4	0.1
virtually fat free, plain	●	2.3	–	25	3.9	0.1
Fruit corner, 125g:						
blueberry	○	19.4	n/a	140	4.6	4.9
strawberry	○	21.4	n/a	148	4.6	4.9
Greek-style, cows, fruit, 1 pot (125g)	○	14	Tr	171	6	10.5
Greek-style, cows, plain, 1 pot (125g)	●	6	–	166	7.1	12.8
Greek-style, sheep, 1 pot (125g)	●	6.3	–	115	6	7.5
Low fat, fruit, 1 pot (125g)	●	17.1	0.4	98	5.3	1.4
Low fat, plain, 1 pot (125g)	●	9.3	–	70	6	1.3
Natural bio yoghurt, 125g	●	7	–	68	5.5	1.9
Orange fat-free bio yoghurt each	●	11.3	0.1	61	5.4	0.2
Raspberry drinking yoghurt, per bottle	○	12.5	0.1	78	2.9	1.8
Soya, fruit, 1 pot (125g)	○	16.1	0.9	91	2.6	2.25
Virtually fat free, fruit, 1 pot (125g)	●	8.78	Tr	59	6	0.3

TIP: Opt for strong-flavoured cheese to add to recipes so that you will need less to get the taste you want.

Food type	GL	Carb (g)	Fibre (g)	Cal (kcal)	Pro (g)	Fat (g)
Virtually fat free, plain, 1 pot (125g)	●	10.3	–	68	6.8	0.3
Yoghurt drink, 125ml:						
natural	●	8.6	n/a	84	6.9	2.4
peach	●	16.2	n/a	94	3.2	1.8
Whole milk, fruit, 1 pot (125g)	●	22.1	–	136	5	3.8
Whole milk, plain, 1 pot (125g)	●	9.8	–	99	7.1	3.8
Butter and Margarine						
Butter:						
lightly salted, 15g		–	n/a	111	–	12.2
spreadable, 15g		Tr	–	112	0.1	12.4
lighter spreadable, 15g		0.1	–	82	0.1	9
Margarine, hard						
animal & vegetable fat, over 80% fat, 15g		0.2	n/a	108	–	11.9
Margarine, soft						
polyunsaturated, over 80% fat, 15g		–	n/a	112	Tr	12.4
Spreads						
Olive oil spread, 15g		0.2	Tr	80	–	8.9

TIP: Mix fruit purée with no- or low-fat Greek yoghurt for a quick fruit fool without the calorie load of double cream.

Food type	GL	Carb (g)	Fibre (g)	Cal (kcal)	Pro (g)	Fat (g)
Olive oil spread, *contd*:						
very low fat (20-25%)		0.4	–	39	0.9	3.8
Polyunsaturated spread:						
buttery, 15g		–	–	80	Tr	8.9
light, 15g		0.9	–	55	–	5.7
low salt, 15g		Tr	–	80	Tr	8.9
sunflower spread, 15g		–	–	95	–	10.5
Pro-biotic, 15g		0.6	Tr	50	–	5.3
light		0.2	Tr	34	0.5	3.5
Cheeses						
Bel Paese, individual, 25g		–	–	77	5.8	6
Bavarian smoked, 25g		0.1	–	69	4.3	5.8
Brie, 25g		0.1	–	76	5.5	6
Caerphilly, 25g		–	–	93	5.8	7.8
Cambozola, 25g		0.1	–	108	3.3	10.5
Camembert, 25g		Tr	–	73	5.4	5.7
Cheddar:						
English, 25g		–	–	104	6.4	8.7
vegetarian, 25g		Tr	–	98	6.4	8
Cheddar-type, half fat, 25g		Tr	–	68	8.2	4

TIP: Don't add butter to spinach. Mix cooked spinach with a little low-fat natural yoghurt instead, then sprinkle with some black pepper and, if you like the taste, a little grated nutmeg.

Food type	GL	Carb (g)	Fibre (g)	Cal (kcal)	Pro (g)	Fat (g)
Cheshire, 25g		–	–	93	5.8	7.8
Cottage cheese:						
plain, 100g	●	3.1	–	101	12.6	4.3
reduced fat, 100g	●	3.3	–	79	13.3	1.5
with additions, 100g	●	2.6	–	95	12.8	3.8
Cream cheese, full fat, 25g		Tr	n/a	110	0.8	11.9
ail & fines herbs, 25g		0.5	–	104	1.8	10.5
au naturel, 25g		0.5	–	106	1.8	10.8
au poivre, 25g		0.5	–	104	1.8	10.5
Danish Blue, 25g		Tr	–	86	5.1	7.2
Dolcelatte, 25g		0.2	–	99	4.3	9
Double Gloucester, 25g		–	–	101	6	8.5
Edam, 25g		Tr	–	85	6.7	6.5
Emmenthal, 25g		0.1	–	93	7.3	7
Feta, 25g		0.4	–	63	3.9	5.1
Goats' milk soft cheese, 25g		0.3	–	80	5.3	6.5
Gorgonzola, 25g		–	–	78	4.8	6.5
Gouda, 25g		Tr	–	94	6.3	7.7
Grana Padano, 25g		–	–	98	8.8	7
Gruyère, 25g		–	–	99	6.8	8
Jarlsberg, 25g		–	–	91	7	7
Lancashire, 25g		–	–	93	5.8	7.8

TIP: Make lassi by beating low-fat natural yoghurt until frothy then diluting it with water. Garnish with a few mint leaves.

Food type	GL	Carb (g)	Fibre (g)	Cal (kcal)	Pro (g)	Fat (g)
Mascarpone, 25g		1.2	–	104	1.2	10.5
Mature cheese, reduced fat, 25g		–	–	77	6.8	5.5
Medium-fat soft cheese, 25g		0.9	–	50	2.5	4.1
Mild cheese, reduced fat, 25g		–	–	77	6.8	5.5
Mozzarella, 25g		–	–	64	4.7	5.1
Parmesan, fresh, 25g		0.2	–	104	9.1	7.4
Quark, 25g		1	–	15	2.8	0.1
Red Leicester, 25g		–	–	101	6	8.5
Ricotta, 25g		0.5	–	34	2.3	2.5
Roquefort, 25g		Tr	–	89	5.8	7.3
Sage Derby, 25g		0.7	–	104	6.1	8.5
Shropshire blue, 25g		0.1	–	92	5.5	7.8
Soft cheese:						
full fat, 25g		0.8	0.1	63	1.5	6
light medium fat, 25g		0.9	0.1	47	2	3.9
light with chives, 25g		0.9	0.1	46	1.9	3.9
light with tomato & basil, 25g	●	1.1	0.1	45	1.9	3.5
Stilton:						
blue, 25g		–	–	103	5.9	8.8
white, 25g		–	–	90	5	7.8
white, with apricots, 25g	●	2	0.4	8	4	6.3
Wensleydale, 25g		–	–	95	5.8	8

TIP: Soya milk is derived from soya beans and retains most of their nutritional value. Choose unsweetened soya milk fortified with calcium.

Food type	GL	Carb (g)	Fibre (g)	Cal (kcal)	Pro (g)	Fat (g)
Wensleydale, *contd:*						
with cranberries, 25g	●	2.3	–	91	5.3	6.8
Cheese Spreads and Processed Cheese						
Cheese spread:						
original, 25g	●	0.9	0.1	62	3.5	5
cheese & chive, 25g	●	1	0.1	59	3.1	4.8
cheese & shrimp, 25g	●	0.7	0.1	59	3.6	4.6
cheese & ham, 25g	●	0.9	0.1	60	3.3	4.8
cheese & garlic, 25g	●	1	–	62	3.9	5
light, 25g	●	1.7	–	43	4	5
Cheese slices:	●					
singles, 25g	●	1.9	0.1	65	3.4	3.6
singles light, 25g	●	1.5	–	51	5	2.8
Cheese triangles, 25g	●	1.5	–	60	2.6	4.9
Processed cheese, plain, 25g	●	1.3	–	74	4.5	5.8
Strip cheese, 25g	●	0.3	–	88	5.4	6.9

TIP: A 25g portion of cheeses, as listed in this section, is a piece about the size of three stacked dice, or the size of your thumb. Sliced or grated, it would be just enough for a modest cheese sandwich. Don't get carried away – check the calorie and fat counts for your favourites.

Food type	GL	Carb (g)	Fibre (g)	Cal (kcal)	Pro (g)	Fat (g)
See also: *Jams, Marmalades and Spreads* For ice cream: *see under Desserts and Puddings*						

TIP: If you're cutting back on dairy, you can boost your calcium intake by eating green leafy vegetables, dried fruit and the kind of oily fish where you eat fine bones – sardines are a good example.

DESSERTS AND PUDDINGS

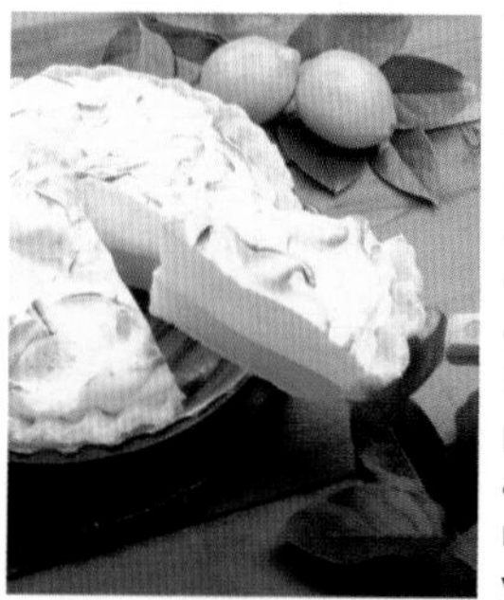

The sea of red dots on these pages should convey the right impression: desserts and puddings are not good news for GL dieters. The exception is ice cream, but the portion you serve is all-important; 100g may well be less than you are used to (about one average scoop). The best thing to do is to combine a little low-GL ice cream with fruit. Tart fruit – like blackcurrants – is best of all, as acidity can reduce overall GI and GL levels. If you are faced with a situation where refusing a dessert is difficult, then take a very small portion. Generally fruit is the best choice, fresh for preference, and many fruit-based recipes can be easily adapted to suit GL eating.

TIP: Cook fresh blackcurrants in a little water until they pop. Stir them well, but don't blend or purée them smooth. Let them cool slightly and then serve with good vanilla ice cream for a delicious, pleasingly tart, hot-and-cold dessert.

Food type	GL	Carb (g)	Fibre (g)	Cal (kcal)	Pro (g)	Fat (g)
Puddings						
Bread pudding, 100g	●	48	n/a	289	5.9	9.5
Christmas pudding, 100g	●	56.3	n/a	329	3	11.8
Creamed rice, 100g	●	16	Tr	93	3.2	2.9
Meringue, 100g	●	96	n/a	381	5.3	Tr
Pavlova, with raspberries, 100g	●	45	Tr	297	2.5	11.9
Profiteroles, 100g	●	18.5	0.4	358	6.2	29.2
Rice pudding, 100g:	●	19.6	0.1	130	4.1	4.3
with sultanas & nutmeg	●	16.6	0.1	105	3.2	2.9
Sago pudding, 100g:						
made with semi-skimmed milk	●	20.1	0.1	93	4	0.2
made with whole milk	●	19.6	0.1	130	4.1	4.3
Semolina pudding, 100g:						
made with semi-skimmed milk	●	20.1	0.1	93	4	0.2
made with whole milk	●	19.6	0.1	130	4.1	4.3
Sponge pudding:						
with chocolate sauce, 100g	●	44.6	1.2	303	5.2	11.5
lemon, 100g	●	50.1	0.6	306	2.7	10.6
treacle, 100g	●	50	0.6	286	2.6	8.4
Spotted Dick, 100g	●	52.7	1	337	3.4	12.6
Tapioca pudding, 100g:						
made with semi-skimmed milk	●	20.1	0.1	93	4	0.2

TIP: A platter of beautifully arranged, perfectly ripe, fresh fruit scattered with a few nuts makes an excellent and GL-friendly finale to a meal.

Food type	GL	Carb (g)	Fibre (g)	Cal (kcal)	Pro (g)	Fat (g)
Tapioca pudding, 100g, *contd:*						
made with whole milk	●	19.6	0.1	130	4.1	4.3
Trifle, 100g	●	21	Tr	166	2.6	8.1
Trifle with fresh cream, 100g	●	19.5	0.5	166	2.4	9.2
Sweet Pies and Flans						
Apple & blackcurrant pies, each	●	35.7	1	227	2.3	8.4
Apple pie, 100g	●	57.8	1.2	384	3.2	15.5
Bakewell tart, 100g	●	56.7	0.9	397	3.8	17.2
cherry bakewell, each	●	28.4	0.7	199	1.8	8.7
Cheesecake, 100g:	●	35.2	1	294	4	16.2
raspberry	●	31.9	0.6	299	4.7	17.2
Custard tart, 100g	●	32.4	–	277	6.3	14.5
Dutch apple tart, 100g	●	34.4	0.6	237	3.2	9.9
Fruit pie, individual:	●	56.7	–	356	4.3	14
pastry top & bottom, 100g	●	33.9	n/a	262	3.1	13.6
wholemeal, one crust, 100g	●	26.5	n/a	185	2.7	8.3
Jam tart, each	●	22.4	0.5	139	1.3	4.9
Lemon meringue pie, 100g	●	43.5	–	251	2.9	8.5
Mince pies, 100g	●	59.9	1.5	395	3.7	15.6
luxury, 100g	●	55.7	1.5	387	3.7	14
Treacle tart, 100g	●	62.8	n/a	379	3.9	14.2

TIP: Push fresh raspberries through a sieve to make a raspberry purée. Spoon over vanilla ice cream, and top with whole fresh raspberries.

Food type	GL	Carb (g)	Fibre (g)	Cal (kcal)	Pro (g)	Fat (g)
Chilled and Frozen Desserts						
Crème brulée, 100g	●	23.5	0.2	251	1.3	17
Crème caramel, 100g	●	20.6	n/a	104	3	1.6
Chocolate nut sundae, 100g	●	26.2	0.2	243	2.6	14.9
Ice cream, 100g:						
Cornish	●	11.3	n/a	92	19	4.4
chocolate	○	11.4	n/a	91	2	4.2
Neapolitan	○	11.8	Tr	83	1.7	3.3
peach melba	○	13.2	n/a	94	1.7	3.8
raspberry ripple	○	13.1	Tr	87	1.6	3.1
strawberry	●	10.5	n/a	84	1.7	3.8
tiramisu	○	15.2	n/a	112	2.1	4.6
vanilla	●	11.0	n/a	87	1.7	4.5
Ice cream bar, chocolate-covered, 100g	●	21.8	Tr	311	5	23.3
Ice cream dessert, frozen, 100g	●	21	Tr	251	3.5	17.6
Instant dessert powder, 100g:						
made up with whole milk	○	14.8	0.2	111	3.1	6.3
Jelly, 100g, *made with water*	●	68.9	n/a	296	5.1	–
Mousse, 100g:						
chocolate	●	19.9	–	149	4	6.5
fruit	●	18	–	143	4.5	6.4

TIP: Toast chopped almonds in a dry frying pan and stir them into no-fat Greek yoghurt. Drizzle a little runny honey over the top.

Food type	GL	Carb (g)	Fibre (g)	Cal (kcal)	Pro (g)	Fat (g)
Sorbet, 100g:						
fruit	●	24.8	1	97	0.2	0.3
lemon	●	32	–	128	–	–
Tiramisu, 100g	●	31.2	0.3	337	3.5	22.2
Vanilla soya dessert, each	●	16.4	1.3	80	3.8	2.3
For yoghurt, *see under Dairy*						
Toppings and Sauces						
Brandy flavour sauce mix, 50ml	●	38.3	–	208	3.1	4.8
Brandy sauce, ready to serve, 50ml	●	8.3	–	49	1.4	0.8
Chocolate custard mix, 50ml:						
chocolate flavour	●	39.3	0.1	208	3.0	4.4
low fat	●	39.3	0.1	203	2.2	4.1
Custard, 50ml:						
made with skimmed milk	●	8.4	Tr	40	1.9	0.1
made with whole milk	●	8.1	n/a	59	2	2.3
canned or carton	●	7	Tr	50	1.5	2
Devon custard, canned, 50ml	●	8	–	51	1.5	1.5
Artificial cream topping, 50ml	●	16.3	0.3	345	3.4	29.3
sugar-free	●	15.3	0.3	348	3.7	30.3

TIP: When it comes to ice cream, the taste of a gourmet brand will be light years better than the supermarket's own-brand economy pack. If you're eating smaller portions, maybe you can afford to splash out.

Food type	GL	Carb (g)	Fibre (g)	Cal (kcal)	Pro (g)	Fat (g)
Maple syrup, organic, 1 tsp	●	4.2	Tr	17	Tr	–
Rum sauce (Bird's), 50ml	●	7.8	–	46	1.4	0.8
White sauce, sweet, 50ml						
made with semi-skimmed milk	●	9.3	n/a	76	2	3.7
made with whole milk	●	9.2	n/a	86	2	4.8

TIP: Try a Caribbean fruit salad for a special dinner party dessert. Cube a melon and a pineapple and slice two mangoes. You could also add a chopped guava and the pulp from a couple of passion fruit. Mix everything together gently and add three tablespoons of white rum. Mix again and serve.

DRINKS

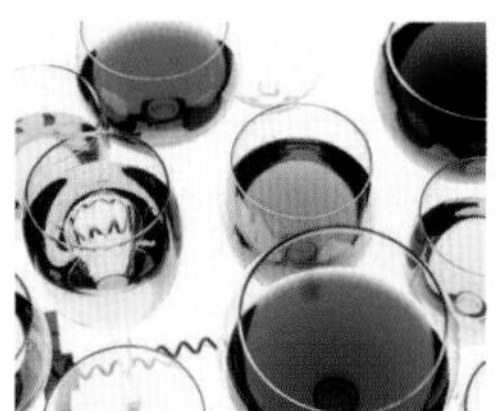

Drinking six to eight glasses of plain water a day is recommended, and some of this liquid can be in the form of herb tea (but not those containing sugar or sweeteners). You may find water tastes better if you add a slice of lemon or lime. Fruit juices, squashes and sports drinks should be avoided on a GL diet, and flavoured mineral waters can be deceptive; check the ingredients closely for hidden sugars. Watch the amount of coffee you drink and moderate it if necessary – get it down to only one cup a day, or stop completely – to reduce the impact of caffeine on insulin levels. Alcoholic drinks are high in sugars though some have a low GL. You will lose weight more rapidly if you stop drinking alcohol during the weight-loss phase of your diet, however, and most GL diets recommend that you do this.

TIP: Most packaged drinks are high in sugars or sugar substitutes, as well as all sorts of flavourings. Check ingredient lists, but as a general principle they are best avoided.

Food type	GL	Carb (g)	Fibre (g)	Cal (kcal)	Pro (g)	Fat (g)
Alcoholic						
Advocaat, 25ml		7.1	–	68	1.2	1.6
Beer, bitter, 500ml:						
canned		11.5	–	160	1.5	Tr
draught		11.5	–	160	1.5	Tr
keg		11.5	–	155	1.5	Tr
Beer, mild draught, 500ml		8.0	–	125	1.0	Tr
Brandy, 25ml		Tr	–	56	Tr	–
Brown ale, bottled, 500ml		15	n/a	150	1.5	–
Cider, 500ml:						
dry		13	n/a	180	Tr	–
sweet		21.5	n/a	210	Tr	–
vintage		36.5	n/a	505	Tr	–
Cognac, 25ml		n/a	n/a	88	n/a	n/a
Gin, 25ml		Tr	–	56	Tr	–
Lager, bottled, 500ml		7.5	–	145	1.0	Tr
Pale ale, bottled, 500ml		10	n/a	140	1.5	Tr
Port, 25ml		3	n/a	39	–	–
Rum, 25ml		Tr	–	56	Tr	–
Sherry, 25ml						
dry		0.4	n/a	29	0.1	–
medium		1.5	n/a	29	–	–

TIP: Sugar is often listed as 'corn syrup' in soft drinks, so watch out for that on labels.

Food type	GL	Carb (g)	Fibre (g)	Cal (kcal)	Pro (g)	Fat (g)
Sherry, *contd*						
sweet	●	1.7	n/a	34	0.1	–
Stout, 500ml:						
bottled	●	21	–	185	1.5	Tr
extra	●	10.5	–	195	1.5	Tr
Strong ale, 500ml	●	30.5	–	360	3.5	Tr
Vermouth, 50ml:						
dry	●	1.5	n/a	55	0.1	–
sweet	●	8.0	n/a	76	Tr	–
bianco	●	n/a	n/a	73	n/a–	n/a
extra dry	●	n/a	n/a	48	n/a	n/a
rosso	●	n/a	n/a	70	n/a	n/a
Vodka, 25ml	●	Tr	–	56	Tr	–
Whisky, 25ml	●	Tr	–	56	Tr	–
Wine, per small glass (125ml):						
red	●	0.3	n/a	85	0.1	–
rosé	●	3.1	n/a	89	0.1	–
white, dry	●	0.8	n/a	83	0.1	–
white, medium	●	3.8	n/a	93	0.1	–
white, sparkling	●	6.4	n/a	93	0.4	–
white, sweet	●	7.4	n/a	118	0.3	–

TIP: Alcohol contains 'empty' calories and can slow down your body's consumption of fat – while your system has alcohol as a source of energy it won't use up other sources, such as body fat.

Food type	GL	Carb (g)	Fibre (g)	Cal (kcal)	Pro (g)	Fat (g)
Liqueurs						
Cherry, 25ml		8.2	–	64	Tr	–
Coffee, 25ml		n/a	n/a	65.5	n/a	–
Coffee cream, 25ml		n/a	n/a	80	n/a	–
Orange, 25ml		n/a	n/a	85	n/a	–
Triple sec, 25ml		n/a	n/a	80	n/a	–
Juices and Cordials						
Apple juice, unsweetened, 250ml		24.8	n/a	95	0.3	0.3
Apple & elderflower juice, 250ml		25.5	n/a	108	1	0.3
Apple & mango juice, 250ml		25.3	n/a	108	1	0.3
Barley water, 250ml:						
lemon, original		54.5	Tr	241	0.8	Tr
no added sugar		27.5	–	28	0.5	–
orange, original		57.8	Tr	244	0.8	Tr
Blackcurrant & apple juice, 250ml		24.3	n/a	108	Tr	Tr
Carrot juice, 250ml		14.3	–	60	1.3	0.3
Cranberry juice, 250ml		29.3	Tr	123	Tr	Tr

TIP: Iced tea makes a refreshing summer drink. Make a pot of good tea, or use herb tea, then strain and chill for an hour. Serve in tall glasses over crushed ice with a slice of lemon and a sprig of mint.

Food type	GL	Carb (g)	Fibre (g)	Cal (kcal)	Pro (g)	Fat (g)
Grape juice, unsweetened, 250ml		29.3	–	115	0.8	0.3
Grapefruit juice, 250ml		22	n/a	103	1.3	Tr
Lemon squash, low calorie, 250ml		1	n/a	18	–	–
Lime juice cordial, undiluted, 25ml		7.5	n/a	28	–	–
Orange & mango fruit juice, no added sugar, 250ml		2	n/a	21	0.5	Tr
Orange & pineapple fruit juice, 250ml		27.5	n/a	120	1.3	Tr
Orange juice, unsweetened, 250ml		22	n/a	90	1.3	0.3
Orange squash, low calorie, 250ml		6	–	25	0.3	–
Pineapple juice, unsweetened, 250ml		26.3	n/a	103	0.8	0.3
Tomato juice, 250ml:		7.5	n/a	35	2	Tr
cocktail (Britvic), 250ml		9	n/a	52	2.3	0.3

TIP: If you want to cut down on the amount of alcohol you drink, start keeping a diary of the number of units you consume. A unit is a small pub measure of wine (125ml), one unit of spirits (25ml) or a half pint (284ml) of lager. Remember that government-recommended totals are 14 units a week for women and 21 a week for men.

Food type	GL	Carb (g)	Fibre (g)	Cal (kcal)	Pro (g)	Fat (g)
Fizzy Drinks						
Apple drink, sparkling, 330ml	●	22.4	n/a	95	Tr	Tr
Bitter lemon, 355ml	●	29.5	n/a	126	Tr	Tr
Cherry Coke, 330ml	●	36.3	n/a	149	–	–
Cherryade, 330ml	●	22.4	n/a	94	Tr	Tr
Cola, 330ml		35	n/a	142	–	–
diet	●	–	n/a	1	–	–
Cream Soda, 330ml	●	17.5	n/a	71	–	–
Dandelion & Burdock, 330ml	●	16.2	n/a	65	Tr	Tr
Ginger Ale, American 330ml	●	30.4	n/a	124	–	–
Ginger Ale, Dry 330ml	●	12.5	n/a	52	–	–
Ginger beer, 330ml	●	28.1	n/a	116	Tr	–
Irn Bru, 330ml	●	33.3	–	135	Tr	Tr
diet, 330ml	●	Tr	–	2	Tr	Tr
Lemon drink, sparkling, 330ml	●	39.6	n/a	165	–	–
low calorie	●	1.3	n/a	7	–	–
Lemonade, 330ml	●	19.1	n/a	73	Tr	–
low calorie		Tr	n/a	5	Tr	Tr
Glucose drink, 330ml	●	59.1	n/a	241	Tr	–
Orange drink, 330ml	●	22.1	n/a	96	Tr	Tr
low calorie	●	2.3	n/a	18	Tr	Tr

TIP: Remember that caffeine can play havoc with your insulin levels. It isn't only found in coffee and tea – cola drinks, including diet colas, are very high in it too.

Food type	GL	Carb (g)	Fibre (g)	Cal (kcal)	Pro (g)	Fat (g)
Ribena, sparkling, 330ml	●	43.9	–	178	–	–
low calorie	●	0.3	–	7	–	–
Tonic water, 330ml	●	20.5	n/a	86	–	–
Water, flavoured, 330ml	●	Tr	–	3	Tr	–
Hot and Milky Drinks						
Beef instant drink, per mug	●	51.3	0.3	425	54.3	0.3
Cappuccino, per sachet:						
instant	●	12	–	72	2	1.7
unsweetened	●	9.8	–	77	2.7	3
Chicken instant drink, per mug	●	48.8	5.3	323	24.3	3.5
Cocoa, per mug						
made with semi-skimmed milk	●	17.4	0.5	142	8.7	4.7
made with whole milk	●	17.0	0.5	190	8.5	10.5
Coffee, black, per mug	●	0.8	n/a	5	0.5	Tr
Coffee creamer, per tsp	●	3.7	–	26	0.2	2.2
virtually fat free, per tsp	●	4.2	–	20	0.1	0.3
Drinking chocolate, per mug						
made with semi-skimmed milk	●	27.3	–	183	9	5
made with whole milk	●	26.8	2.5	225	8.8	10
Espresso, per 100ml	●	10	11.5	104	15.2	0.4

TIP: If you know that you'll find restricting the amount of alcohol you drink difficult, then it's best to cut it out completely as you diet down to your target weight. The weight will drop off much faster.

Food type	GL	Carb (g)	Fibre (g)	Cal (kcal)	Pro (g)	Fat (g)
Herb teas, per mug	●	–	–	–	0.1	–
Ice tea, per mug	●	16.8	n/a	70	–	–
Malted milk, per mug						
made with semi-skimmed milk	●	71.3	1.8	460	23.5	11.5
made with whole milk	●	70.8	1.8	575	23	22.8
Malted milk light,						
made with water, per mug	●	57.8	1.5	290	11.8	3.0
Strawberry milkshake, 250ml						
made with semi-skimmed milk	●	62.2	–	387	17	8.5
made with whole milk	●	47.2	–	420	17	19.5
Tea, black, per cup	●	Tr	n/a	Tr	0.3	Tr

TIP: A tablespoon or so of a liqueur like Grand Marnier or Cointreau on a fruit salad can give it a delicious flavour and avoid the need to use fruit syrups or juices.

EGGS

Eggs are carb-free but the cholesterol they contain has led some dietitians to suggest they should only be eaten infrequently, or that only the whites should be used. However, recent research has found that one egg a day is perfectly healthy for most people. Should you decide to incorporate eggs in your diet – and they are rich in nutrients and a great source of B vitamins and vitamin E – then opt for organic, free range or omega-3 enriched ones. Consider your cooking methods too; boiled or poached eggs are a better choice than fried, for example.

TIP: Farmers' markets can be a good source of eggs, but it's worth sticking to organic. Other eggs will taste fishy or bland once you've become accustomed to golden-yolked organic ones.

Food type	GL	Carb (g)	Fibre (g)	Cal (kcal)	Pro (g)	Fat (g)
Eggs, chicken, 1 medium:						
raw, whole		Tr	–	78	6.5	5.8
raw, white only		Tr	n/a	17	4.3	Tr
raw, yolk only		Tr	n/a	59	2.8	5.3
boiled		Tr	n/a	76	6.5	5.6
fried, in vegetable oil		Tr	n/a	93	7.1	7.2
poached		Tr	n/a	76	6.5	5.6
Eggs, duck, raw, whole		Tr	n/a	84	7.4	6.1
Omelette (2 eggs, 10g butter):						
plain	●	–	n/a	228	12.7	19.6
with 25g cheese	●	Tr	n/a	475	27.9	40.3
Scrambled (2 eggs with 15 ml milk, 20g butter)	●	0.8	n/a	310	13.1	28.2

TIP: It is easiest to peel hard-boiled eggs if the eggs are a few days old. Really fresh ones are difficult to peel as the white adheres to the shell much more strongly.

FISH AND SEAFOOD

Fish should be included in your diet at least twice or three times a week. White fish is an excellent source of protein without a high fat load, and oily fish like salmon or tuna are high in omega-3 fatty acids which are vital for many aspects of health. Shellfish can be high in cholesterol, so you may want to save them for special occasions. Fish only has a GL value if it has been treated – coated in breadcrumbs or batter, for example, or served with a sauce. Avoid coatings completely, and be careful with sauces.

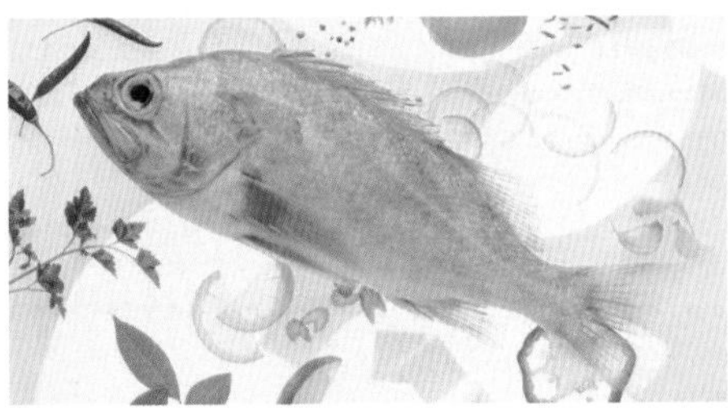

TIP: Cooking fish in foil helps to eliminate fishy smells. Wrap pieces of cod loin in foil, with chopped spring onion, slices of fresh ginger, a squeeze of lemon juice and a little shoyu soy sauce. Seal the parcel well and bake in the oven at 200°C/gas mark 6 for about 15 minutes, depending on the thickness of the fish.

Food type	GL	Carb (g)	Fibre (g)	Cal (kcal)	Pro (g)	Fat (g)
Fish and Seafood						
Anchovies, in oil,						
drained, 100g		–	–	191	25.2	10
Cockles, boiled, 100g		Tr	n/a	53	12	0.6
Cod:						
baked fillets, 100g		Tr	n/a	96	21.4	1.2
dried, salted, boiled, 100g		–	n/a	138	32.5	0.9
in batter, fried, 100g		11.7	n/a	247	16.1	15.4
in crumbs, fried, 100g		15.2	n/a	235	12.4	14.3
in parsley sauce, boiled, 100g		2.8	n/a	84	12	2.8
poached fillets, 100g		Tr	n/a	94	20.9	1.1
steaks, grilled, 100g		Tr	n/a	95	20.8	1.3
Cod roe, hard, fried, 100g		3	n/a	202	20.9	11.9
Coley fillets, steamed, 100g		–	n/a	105	23.3	1.3
Crab						
boiled, 100g		Tr	n/a	128	19.5	5.5
canned, 100g		Tr	n/a	77	18.1	0.5
dressed, 100g		n/a	n/a	105	16.9	14.2
Eels, jellied, 100g		Tr	n/a	98	8.4	7.1
Haddock:						
in crumbs, fried, 100g		12.6	n/a	196	14.7	10

TIP: Tinned tuna is a useful storecupboard standby. Always buy it in brine or spring water, and rinse before use to reduce salt levels. For a tasty tuna dip, blend it with low-fat cream cheese and a little paprika.

Food type	GL	Carb (g)	Fibre (g)	Cal (kcal)	Pro (g)	Fat (g)
Haddock, *contd*:						
smoked, steamed, 100g		–	n/a	101	23.3	0.9
steamed, 100g		–	n/a	89	20.9	0.6
Halibut, grilled, 100g		–	n/a	121	25.3	2.2
Herring:						
fried, 100g	●	1.5	–	234	23.1	15.1
grilled, 100g		–	–	199	20.4	13
Kippers, grilled, 100g		–	n/a	255	20.1	19.4
Lemon sole:						
steamed, 100g		–	n/a	91	20.6	0.9
goujons, baked, 100g	●	14.7	n/a	187	16	14.6
goujons, fried, 100g	●	14.3	n/a	374	15.5	28.7
Lobster, boiled, 100g		–	–	119	22.1	3.4
Mackerel, grilled, 100g		–	n/a	239	20.8	17.3
Mussels, boiled, 100g		Tr	–	87	17.2	2
Pilchards,						
canned in tomato sauce, 100g	●	0.7	Tr	126	18.8	5.4
Plaice						
in batter, fried, 100g	●	12	–	257	15.2	16.8
in crumbs, fried, 100g	●	8.6	–	228	18	13.7
goujons, baked, 100g	●	27.7	–	304	8.8	18.3

TIP: Don't serve a rich hollandaise sauce with salmon. Instead try finely chopped cucumber or spring onion, mixed with equal measures of no-fat Greek yoghurt and low-fat mayo.

Food type	GL	Carb (g)	Fibre (g)	Cal (kcal)	Pro (g)	Fat (g)
Plaice, *contd:*						
goujons, fried, 100g	●	27	–	426	8.5	32.3
steamed, 100g		–	–	93	18.9	1.9
Prawns: *shelled, boiled*, 100g		–	n/a	99	22.6	0.9
boiled, weighed in shells, 175g		–	–	72	15.1	1.2
king prawns, freshwater, 100g		–	n/a	70	16.8	0.3
North Atlantic, peeled, 100g		–	–	99	22.6	0.9
tiger king, cooked, 100g		–	n/a	61	13.5	0.6
Roe:						
cod, hard, fried, 100g	●	3	n/a	202	20.9	11.9
herring, soft, fried, 100g	●	4.7	–	244	21.1	15.8
Salmon:						
pink, canned in brine,						
drained, 100g		–	n/a	153	23.5	6.6
grilled steak, 100g		–	n/a	215	24.2	13.1
smoked, 100g		–	n/a	142	25.4	4.5
steamed, flesh only, 100g		–	n/a	194	21.8	11.9
Sardines:						
canned in oil, drained, 100g		–	n/a	220	23.3	14.1
canned in tomato sauce, 100g	●	1.4	n/a	162	17	9.9
Scampi tails, premium, 100g	○	26	n/a	230	8.4	10.9

TIP: Anchovies are one of the oily fishes, related to herrings. Always drain them of their oil and blot dry on kitchen paper before use.They can add a useful burst of flavour to a salad or dressing.

Food type	GL	Carb (g)	Fibre (g)	Cal (kcal)	Pro (g)	Fat (g)
Shrimps:						
canned, drained, 100g		Tr	n/a	94	20.8	1.2
frozen, without shells, 100g		Tr	n/a	73	16.5	0.8
Skate, fried in butter, 100g	●	4.9	0.2	199	17.9	12.1
Sole: *see* Lemon sole						
Swordfish, grilled, 100g	●	–	n/a	139	22.9	5.2
Trout:						
brown, steamed, 100g		–	–	135	23.5	4.5
rainbow, grilled, 100g		–	n/a	135	21.5	5.4
Tuna, fresh, grilled, 100g		0.4	–	170	24.3	7.9
canned in brine, 100g		–	n/a	99	23.5	0.6
canned in oil, 100g		–	n/a	189	27.1	9
Whelks, boiled,						
weighed with shells, 100g		Tr	n/a	89	19.5	1.2
Whitebait, fried, 100g	●	5.3	n/a	525	19.5	47.5
Whiting:						
steamed, flesh only, 100g		–	n/a	92	20.9	0.9
in crumbs, fried, 100g	●	7	n/a	191	18.1	10.3
Winkles, boiled,						
weighed with shells, 100g		Tr	n/a	72	15.4	1.2

TIP: Fish cooks much more quickly than most meats, making it an excellent choice for anyone in a hurry; in fact, overcooking spoils it. Grill fish, or poach it in skimmed milk flavoured with a bay leaf and a little lemon rind; don't be tempted to fry it when you're dieting.

Food type	GL	Carb (g)	Fibre (g)	Cal (kcal)	Pro (g)	Fat (g)
Breaded, Battered or in Sauces						
Calamari in batter, 100g	○	13	1.5	177	7.8	10.4
Fish cakes, 100g						
fried, each	○	16.8	n/a	218	8.6	13.4
Fish fingers						
fried in oil, 100g	○	17.2	0.6	233	13.5	12.7
grilled, 100g	○	19.3	0.7	214	15.1	9
oven crispy, 100g	○	17	0.5	236	10.5	14
Fish steaks in butter sauce, 100g	●	3.2	0.1	84	9.1	3.9
Fish steaks in parsley sauce, 100g	●	3.1	0.1	82	9.1	3.7
Kipper fillets with butter, 100g		–	–	205	15	16
Prawn Cocktail (Lyons), 100g	●	4.5	n/a	429	5.7	42.9
Seafood sticks, 100g	●	14.5	1	95	8.1	0.4
Shrimps, potted, 100g		–	–	358	16.5	32.4

TIP: Fruit and fish can complement each other very successfully. Pink grapefruit and smoked salmon go well, mango works beautifully with smoked fish, and an anchovy and melon salad makes an unusual starter. Cut the melon into cubes, and chop the well-drained anchovies (soak them in milk for a while if they seem too salty). Combine and sprinkle with a little orange and lemon juice.

FRUIT

All fruit contains fructose, the naturally occurring fruit sugar, but that doesn't mean you can't eat it on a GL diet. Always eat the whole fruit rather than the juice, and eat the peel if it's edible as the fibre slows down the process of digestion significantly. Pesticide residues can be a problem so wash fruit thoroughly and choose seasonal organic fruit for preference. Some dried fruits are high GL so be careful; apricots are probably the best bet. Tinned fruit often contains added sugars and should be avoided.

TIP: Avocado goes well with citrus fruit. Peel and slice two avocados, and sprinkle with lemon juice. Skin a grapefruit and an orange, taking care to remove as much pith as possible. Interleave the orange and grapefruit slices with slices of avocado, sprinkle with black pepper and serve as a starter.

Food type	GL	Carb (g)	Fibre (g)	Cal (kcal)	Pro (g)	Fat (g)
Apple, 1 medium	●	20.4	n/a	82	0.7	0.2
Apples, stewed						
with sugar (60g)	○	11.5	n/a	44	0.2	0.1
without sugar (60g)	●	4.9	n/a	20	0.2	0.1
Apricots: 1 fresh	○	3.7	n/a	16	0.5	0.1
dried, 8 halves	●	9.9	1.7	45	1.1	0.2
canned in juice, 100g	○	8.4	n/a	34	0.5	0.1
canned in syrup, 100g	○	16.1	n/a	63	0.4	0.1
Avocado, half medium	●	1.6	n/a	160	1.6	16.4
Banana, 1 medium	○	23.2	n/a	95	1.2	0.3
Blackberries:						
fresh, 75g	●	3.8	n/a	19	0.7	0.2
stewed with sugar, 75g	○	10.4	n/a	42	0.5	0.2
stewed without sugar, 75g	●	3.3	4.2	16	0.6	0.2
Blackcurrants:						
fresh, 75g	●	5	n/a	21	0.7	Tr
stewed with sugar, 75g	○	11.3	n/a	44	0.5	Tr
canned in syrup, 75g	○	13.8	2.7	54	0.5	Tr
Blueberries, fresh, 75g	●	7.6	1.6	32	0.4	0.2
Cherries, half cup fresh (90g)	●	10.4	0.8	43	0.8	0.09
Cherries, *glacé*, 25g	○	16.6	0.2	63	0.1	–

TIP: Acid reduces the overall GI/GL value of a dish, so use lemon juice liberally. If you can, buy unwaxed organic lemons, as pesticide residues can easily penetrate the skin of citrus fruit.

Food type	GL	Carb (g)	Fibre (g)	Cal (kcal)	Pro (g)	Fat (g)
Clementines, 1 medium	●	6.6	0.9	28	0.7	0.1
Coconut:						
creamed, 2 tbsp	●	1.4	n/a	134	1.2	13.8
desiccated, 2 tbsp	●	1.3	n/a	121	1.1	12.4
milk, 100ml	●	1.6	–	166	1.6	17.0
Cranberries, fresh, 75g	●	3	3.2	12	–	–
Damsons:						
fresh, 75g	●	7.2	n/a	29	0.4	Tr
stewed with sugar (2 tbsp)	●	5.7	n/a	22	0.1	Tr
Dates, quarter cup (50g)	●	15.7	n/a	62	0.8	0.1
Figs:						
1 fresh	●	9.6	1.7	37	0.4	0.2
dried, ready to eat, 50g	●	24.5	0.8	112	1.7	0.8
canned in syrup, 100g	●	18	0.7	75	0.4	0.1
Fruit cocktail, 100g						
canned in juice	●	7.2	n/a	29	0.4	Tr
canned in syrup	●	14.8	n/a	57	0.4	Tr
Gooseberries:						
fresh, 75g	●	2.3	n/a	14	0.8	0.3
stewed with sugar (2 tbsp)	●	3.9	n/a	16	0.2	0.1
Grapefruit, half, fresh	●	7.7	n/a	34	0.9	0.1

TIP: Make an attractive fruit salad using cubed watermelon, black seedless grapes, a little Grand Marnier and a squeeze of lemon juice. Chill for an hour before serving, stirring occasionally during this time.

Food type	**GL**	**Carb (g)**	**Fibre (g)**	**Cal (kcal)**	**Pro (g)**	**Fat (g)**
Grapes, black/white, seedless,						
fresh, 75g	●	11.6	n/a	45	0.3	0.1
Greengages:						
fresh, 75g	●	6.5	1.2	26	0.4	Tr
stewed with sugar (2 tbsp)	○	8	0.4	32	0.4	–
Guavas, fresh, 60g	●	3	n/a	16	0.5	0.3
Honeydew melon: *see* Melon						
Jackfruit, fresh, 75g	●	16.1	–	66	1.0	0.2
Kiwi fruit, peeled, each	●	10.6	n/a	49	1.1	0.5
Lemon, whole	●	3.2	n/a	19	1	0.3
Lychees, fresh, 75g	●	10.7	n/a	44	0.7	0.1
canned in syrup, 100g	○	17.7	n/a	68	0.4	Tr
Mandarin oranges, 100g:						
canned in juice	●	7.7	n/a	32	0.7	Tr
canned in syrup	○	13.4	n/a	52	0.5	Tr
Mangos, 1 medium	●	16.3	n/a	66	0.8	0.2
Melon, fresh, medium slice:						
cantaloupe	●	4.9	n/a	22	0.7	0.1
galia	●	6.3	n/a	27	0.6	0.1
honeydew	●	7.5	n/a	32	0.7	0.1
watermelon	●	8	n/a	35	0.6	0.3

TIP: Berries have so little carbohydrate that their GL is difficult to measure, so eat them as often as you wish. They are high in fibre, and blackcurrants and strawberries are excellent sources of vitamin C.

Food type	GL	Carb (g)	Fibre (g)	Cal (kcal)	Pro (g)	Fat (g)
Nectarines, 1 medium		13.5	n/a	60	2.1	0.1
Oranges, 1 medium		12.9	n/a	56	1.7	0.2
Papaya, half, fresh		10	n/a	41	0.6	0.1
Passionfruit, 75g						
fresh (flesh & pips only)		4.4	n/a	27	2	0.3
Paw-paw, half, fresh		10	2.5	41	0.6	0.1
Peach, 1 medium		11.5	n/a	50	1.5	0.2
canned in juice, 100g		9.7	n/a	39	0.6	Tr
canned in syrup, 100g		14	n/a	55	0.5	Tr
Pear, 1 medium		15	n/a	60	0.5	0.2
canned in juice, 100g		8.5	n/a	33	0.3	Tr
canned in syrup, 100g		13.2	n/a	50	0.2	Tr
Pineapple, fresh, 60g		6.1	n/a	25	0.2	0.1
canned in juice, 100g		12.2	n/a	47	0.3	Tr
canned in syrup, 100g		16.5	n/a	64	0.5	Tr
Plums, 1 medium		8.8	n/a	36	0.6	0.1
Prunes, canned in juice, 100g		19.7	n/a	79	0.7	0.2
canned in syrup, 100g		23	n/a	90	0.6	0.2
Prunes, dried: *see under* Snacks						
Raisins: *see under* Snacks						
Raspberries, fresh, 60g		2.8	n/a	15	0.8	0.2

TIP: Oranges are high in vitamin C, but are also rich in vitamins A, B1 and folic acid. Don't be tempted just to drink the juice as you'd miss out on useful fibre.

Food type	GL	Carb (g)	Fibre (g)	Cal (kcal)	Pro (g)	Fat (g)
Rhubarb, fresh, raw, 60g	●	0.5	n/a	4	0.5	0.1
stewed with sugar (2 tbsp)	●	3.4	n/a	14	0.3	–
stewed without sugar (2 tbsp)	●	0.2	0.4	2	0.3	–
Satsumas, 1 medium	●	12.8	n/a	54	1.4	0.2
Strawberries, 70g	●	4.2	n/a	19	0.6	0.1
Tangerines, fresh, one	●	8	n/a	35	0.9	0.1
Watermelon, *see under* Melon						

TIP: For a delicious fruit salad try a mix of black- and redcurrants in Cointreau. Mix 2 tablespoons Cointreau with some grated orange rind, a squeeze of orange juice and a teaspoon of honey. Put 250g each of black- and redcurrants in a serving bowl and pour the Cointreau mixture over; stir well but gently. Chill in the fridge overnight.

JAMS, MARMALADES AND SPREADS

Most jams and marmalades have acceptable GL levels, providing you adhere to the portion sizes. There is a wider range of nutrients in savoury spreads and nut butters, but once again portion control is important, particularly bearing in mind the high calorie content of many nut butters. If you decide you want to eat jams or marmalades, read labels carefully and don't buy those brands where the first listed ingredient is sugar: remember, ingredients are listed in descending order of volume.

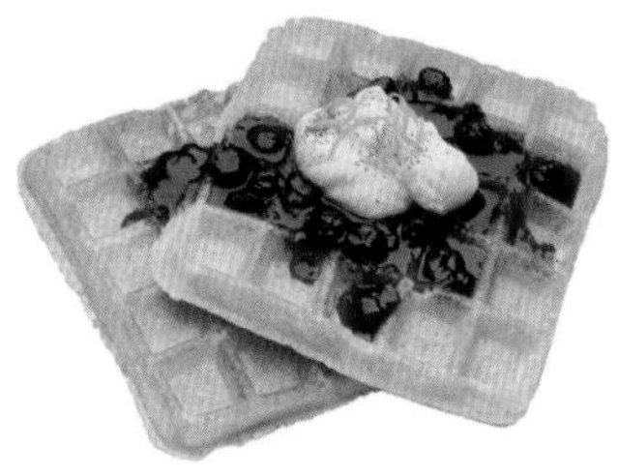

TIP: Marmite is a great source of B vitamins, but most people only use it on toast. A little added to a casserole or soup will give a delicious deeper flavour; just be careful to keep it to a small amount.

Food type	GL	Carb (g)	Fibre (g)	Cal (kcal)	Pro (g)	Fat (g)
Jams and Marmalades						
Apricot conserve, 1 tsp	●	3.2	–	13	–	–
Apricot fruit spread, 1 tsp:						
diet	●	1.5	–	6	–	–
organic	●	1.7	0.1	7	–	Tr
Apricot jam, 1 tsp:						
reduced sugar	●	2.3	n/a	9	–	–
sucrose free	●	3.2	n/a	13	–	Tr
Blackcurrant jam, 1 tsp:						
reduced sugar	●	2.3	n/a	9	–	–
sucrose free	●	3.4	n/a	13	–	Tr
Blueberry & blackberry jam,			–		–	–
organic, 1 tsp	●	3	0.1	13	–	–
Grapefruit fruit spread, 1 tsp	●	1.9	0.1	7	–	–
Grapefruit marmalade, 1 tsp	●	3.1	n/a	12	–	–
Honey, 1 tsp:						
clear	●	3.7	n/a	15	–	Tr
honeycomb	●	3.6	n/a	14	–	0.2
set	●	3.5	–	14	–	–
Lemon curd, 1 tsp	●	3.1	–	14	–	0.2
Marmalade:						
orange, 1 tsp	●	2.1	n/a	8	–	–

TIP: Stone some black olives and whizz them in a blender or food processor to make a tapenade – delicious spread on oatcakes.

Food type	GL	Carb (g)	Fibre (g)	Cal (kcal)	Pro (g)	Fat (g)
Marmalade, *contd:*						
Dundee, 1 tsp	●	2.7	–	11	–	–
organic, 1 tsp	●	3.2	–	13	–	–
thick-cut, 1 tsp	●	3.5	–	13	–	–
Morello cherry fruit spread						
organic, 1 tsp	●	1.7	0.1	7	–	Tr
Pineapple & ginger fruit						
spread, 1 tsp	●	1.9	0.1	7	–	Tr
Raspberry conserve, 1 tsp	●	3.2	–	13	–	–
Raspberry fruit spread, 1 tsp:						
diet	●	1.5	–	6	–	–
organic	●	1.7	0.1	7	–	Tr
Raspberry jam, 1 tsp:	●	3	n/a	12	–	–
organic	●	3.2	–	13	–	–
reduced sugar	●	2.3	n/a	9	–	–
sucrose free	●	3.2	n/a	13	–	–
Rhubarb & ginger jam,						
reduced sugar, 1 tsp	●	2.5	–	10	–	Tr
Seville orange fruit spread, 1 tsp						
reduced sugar	●	1.5	–	6	–	–
organic	●	1.7	0.1	7	–	Tr

TIP: Even though most jams and marmalades are low GL, remember that this depends on the quantity you use. Keep to a teaspoonful and spread it thinly.

Food type	GL	Carb (g)	Fibre (g)	Cal (kcal)	Pro (g)	Fat (g)
Strawberry fruit spread, 1 tsp	●	1.4	–	6	–	–
organic	●	1.7	0.1	7	–	Tr
Strawberry jam, 1 tsp:						
classic	●	3	n/a	12	–	–
reduced sugar	●	2.3	n/a	9	–	–
sucrose free	●	3.2	n/a	13	–	Tr
Wild blackberry jelly, *reduced sugar*, 1 tsp	●	2.7	0.1	11	–	–
Wild blueberry fruit spread, *organic*, 1 tsp	●	1.8	0.2	7	–	–
Nut Butters						
Almond butter, 1 tsp	●	0.3	0.4	31	1.3	2.8
Cashew butter, 1 tsp	●	0.9	0.2	32	1.2	2.6
Chocolate nut spread, 1 tsp	●	3.1	n/a	28	0.3	1.7
Hazelnut butter, 1 tsp	●	0.3	0.3	34	0.8	3.3
Peanut butter, 1 tsp:						
crunchy	●	0.8	0.3	30	1.2	2.5
smooth	●	0.7	n/a	30	1.3	2.4
organic	●	0.6	0.3	30	1.5	2.4
stripy chocolate	●	1.7	0.2	31	0.7	2.3
Tahini paste, 1 tsp	●	–	n/a	30	0.9	2.9

TIP: Don't forget about calories. Nut butters may have a low GL, but they are high in calories when compared to the same quantity of jam.

Food type	GL	Carb (g)	Fibre (g)	Cal (kcal)	Pro (g)	Fat (g)
Savoury Spreads and Pastes						
Beef spread, 1 tsp	●	0.1	n/a	10	0.9	0.7
Cheese spread, 1 tsp:	●	0.4	–	10	n/a	0.7
reduced fat	●	0.4	–	9	0.8	0.5
very low fat	●	0.4	0.1	6	0.9	0.1
See also under: Dairy						
Chicken spread, 1 tsp	●	0.1	n/a	11	0.7	0.9
Crab spread, 1 tsp	●	0.1	n/a	5	0.8	0.2
Fish paste, 1 tsp	●	0.2	n/a	8	0.7	0.5
Guacamole, 1 tsp:						
reduced fat	●	0.4	n/a	7	n/a	0.6
Hummus, 1 tsp	●	0.6	n/a	9	0.4	0.6
Liver pâté, 1 tsp:	●	–	n/a	17	0.6	1.6
low-fat	●	0.2	Tr	10	0.9	0.6
Meat paste, 1 tsp	●	0.2	–	4	0.8	0.6
Mushroom pâté, 1 tsp	●	0.4	–	12	0.4	0.9
Salmon spread, 1 tsp	●	0.2	–	9	0.7	0.5
Sandwich spread, 1 tsp	●	1.3	–	11	0.1	0.6

TIP: Diabetic and reduced-sugar jams might seem tempting, but double-check the ingredients. Aspartame – a sugar substitute – has had a bad press in recent years, with some researchers linking it to an increased risk of developing heart disease and certain cancers. And many low-sugar jams contain polyols like maltitol or mannitol, which can have a surprisingly laxative effect.

Food type	GL	Carb (g)	Fibre (g)	Cal (kcal)	Pro (g)	Fat (g)
Sandwich spread, *contd:*						
cucumber, 1 tsp	●	1	–	9	0.1	0.6
Taramasalata, 1 tsp	●	0.2	n/a	25	0.2	2.6
Toast toppers, 1 tsp:	●					
chicken & mushroom	●	0.3	–	3	0.3	0.1
ham & cheese	●	0.4	–	5	0.4	0.2
Tzatziki, 1 tsp	●	0.2	n/a	6	0.4	0.5
Yeast extract, half tsp	●	0.9	0.2	11	1.9	–

TIP: If you hanker after garlic bread, make the Tuscan version, *fettunta:* rub a slice of toasted sourdough bread with a clove of garlic and then drizzle on a little good olive oil.

MEAT AND POULTRY

There are no carbs in meat or poultry unless it has been processed. Be circumspect about all processed meats, like sausages or deli meats. Some meats have high levels of fat and are high in calories. (Patrick Holford's diet does not allow red meat at all during the weight-loss phase.) If you do eat meat, make sure you remove as much visible fat as you can and don't add more during cooking. Organic meat is expensive but portion control means you'll be eating comparatively less; it may be worth it.

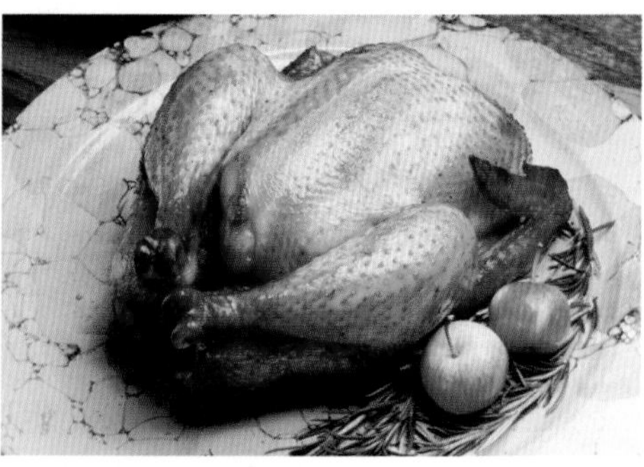

TIP: Chopped fresh herbs can be frozen in ice cube trays filled with water; just drop a couple of cubes into a casserole when you want to use them.

Food type	GL	Carb (g)	Fibre (g)	Cal (kcal)	Pro (g)	Fat (g)
Cooked Meats						
Bacon, 3 rashers, back (50g):						
dry fried		–	n/a	148	12.1	11
grilled		–	n/a	144	11.6	10.8
microwaved		–	n/a	154	12.1	11.7
Bacon, 3 rashers, middle (50g),						
grilled		–	n/a	154	12.4	11.6
Bacon, 3 rashers, streaky (50g):						
fried		–	n/a	168	11.9	13.3
grilled		–	n/a	169	11.9	13.5
Beef, 100g:						
roast rib		–	n/a	300	29.1	20.4
mince, stewed		–	–	209	21.8	13.5
rump steak, lean, grilled		–	–	177	31	5.9
rump steak, lean, fried		–	–	183	30.9	6.6
sausages, see under Sausages						
silverside, lean only, boiled		–	n/a	184	30.4	6.9
stewing steak, stewed		–	n/a	203	29.2	9.6
topside, lean only, roasted		–	n/a	202	36.2	6.3
topside, lean & fat, roasted		–	n/a	244	32.8	12.5
Beef grillsteaks, grilled,						
100g		0.5	n/a	305	22.1	23.9

TIP: Lean beef is low in fat (and saturates), and is a great source of protein, B vitamins and iron.

Food type	GL	Carb (g)	Fibre (g)	Cal (kcal)	Pro (g)	Fat (g)
Burgers, each:						
beefburgers (100g) *fried*		0.1	n/a	329	28.5	23.9
beefburgers (100g) *grilled*		0.1	n/a	326	26.5	24.4
quarter-pounder (120g)	●	6.1	0.5	305	17.5	23.4
chicken burger	●	10	0.5	140	7.5	7.9
vegetable burger	●	27.7	2.3	238	3.1	12.7
vegetable quarter-pounder	●	33.6	2.5	288	6.5	14.4
Black pudding, 2 slices, fried	●	29	n/a	519	18	37.6
Chicken, 100g:						
breast, grilled		–	n/a	148	32	2.2
breast in crumbs, fried	●	14.8	n/a	242	18	12.7
breast, stir fried		–	n/a	161	29.7	4.6
1 drumstick, roast		–	n/a	185	25.8	9.1
1 leg quarter, roast (175g)		–	n/a	413	36.6	29.6
light & dark meat, roasted		–	n/a	177	27.3	7.5
light meat, roasted		–	n/a	153	30.2	3.6
Duck, 100g:						
crispy, Chinese style		0.3	–	331	27.9	24.2
meat only, roasted		–	n/a	195	25.3	10.4
meat, fat & skin, roasted		–	n/a	423	20	38.1

TIP: Don't thicken meat juices with flour to make gravy. Put the roasting dish over an oven ring, add a slug of red wine or sherry and cook at a high temperature, stirring all the while. It will be thinner than your normal gravy, but will also have a delicious flavour.

Food type	GL	Carb (g)	Fibre (g)	Cal (kcal)	Pro (g)	Fat (g)
Gammon, joint, boiled, 100g		–	n/a	204	23.3	12.3
Gammon, rashers, grilled, 100g		–	n/a	199	27.5	9.9
Goose, roasted, 100g		–	n/a	301	27.5	21.2
Haggis, boiled, 100g	●	19.2	n/a	310	10.7	21.7
Kidney, lamb, fried, 100g		–	n/a	188	23.7	10.3
Lamb, 100g:						
breast, lean only, roasted		–	n/a	273	26.7	18.5
breast, lean & fat, roasted		–	n/a	359	22.4	29.9
cutlets, lean only, grilled		–	n/a	238	28.5	13.8
cutlets, lean & fat, grilled		–	n/a	367	24.5	29.9
loin chops, lean only, grilled		–	n/a	213	29.2	10.7
loin chops, lean & fat, grilled		–	n/a	305	26.5	22.1
leg, lean only, roasted		–	n/a	203	29.7	9.4
leg, lean & fat, roasted		–	–	240	28.1	14.2
mince, stewed		–	n/a	208	24.4	12.3
stewed		–	n/a	240	26.6	14.8
shoulder, lean only, roasted		–	n/a	218	27.2	12.1
shoulder, lean & fat, roasted		–	n/a	298	24.7	22.1
Liver, calf, fried, 100g		Tr	n/a	176	22.3	9.6
Liver, chicken, fried, 100g		Tr	n/a	169	22.1	8.9

TIP: Instead of using sugary chutneys with Indian food, opt for yoghurt and cucumber raita or marinated raw onion. Mix thinly sliced onion rings with lemon juice, black pepper and salt; leave to marinate for an hour and then transfer the onion to a serving dish.

Food type	GL	Carb (g)	Fibre (g)	Cal (kcal)	Pro (g)	Fat (g)
Liver, lamb, fried, 100g		Tr	n/a	237	30.1	12.9
Oxtail, stewed, 100g		–	n/a	243	30.5	13.4
Pheasant, roasted, 100g		–	n/a	220	27.9	12
Pork, 100g:						
belly rashers, grilled		–	n/a	320	27.4	23.4
loin chops, lean, grilled		–	n/a	184	31.6	6.4
leg, lean only, roasted		–	–	182	33	5.5
leg, lean & fat, roasted		–	–	215	30.9	10.2
steaks		–	n/a	198	32.4	7.6
Pork sausages: *see* Sausages						
Rabbit, meat only, stewed, 100g		–	n/a	114	21.2	3.2
Sausages:						
beef sausages (2), grilled		14.7	0.8	313	15	22
Cumberland sausages (2)		9.8	1	215	9.9	15.2
Frankfurters (2)		2.3	Tr	369	14.1	33.8
Lincolnshire sausages (2)		18	1.3	345	14.6	23.9
pork sausages (2), fried		11.2	n/a	347	15.7	26.9
Saveloy, 100g		10.8	n/a	296	13.8	22.3
Tongue, fat & skin removed, *stewed*, 100g		–	–	289	18.2	24
Tripe, dressed, 100g		–	n/a	33	7.1	0.5

TIP: Many meat products from deli counters are either high in fat or have had sugar, colourings and/or starchy fillers added.

Food type	GL	Carb (g)	Fibre (g)	Cal (kcal)	Pro (g)	Fat (g)
Turkey, 100g:						
breast fillet, grilled		–	n/a	155	35	1.7
dark meat, roasted		–	n/a	177	29.4	6.6
light meat, roasted		–	n/a	153	33.7	2
Veal, escalope, fried, 100g		–	–	196	33.7	6.8
Venison, haunch, meat only, *roasted*, 100g		–	n/a	165	35.6	2.5
White pudding, 100g	●	36.3	n/a	450	7	31.8
Cold Meats						
Beef, roasted, 50g						
silverside	●	1.2	Tr	69	9.6	2.9
topside	●	0.2	n/a	79	12.5	3
Chicken, roasted breast meat, 50g		0.1	Tr	76	13.5	2.4
Chorizo, 50g	●	2	–	194	11.5	15.5
Corned beef, 50g	●	0.5	n/a	103	13	5.5
Garlic sausage, 50g	●	2.9	0.3	95	7.7	5.8
Ham & pork, chopped, 50g	●	0.7	0.2	138	7.2	11.8
Ham, 50g:						
canned		1	Tr	82	6	6
honey-roast	●	1.5	–	70	11	2.2

TIP: Choose back bacon rather than streaky and trim off the fat before cooking. Grill or dry-fry bacon to avoid adding more fat.

Food type	GL	Carb (g)	Fibre (g)	Cal (kcal)	Pro (g)	Fat (g)
Ham, *contd*:						
mustard	●	0.9	–	62	11.5	1.3
on the bone	●	0.4	0.4	68	10.5	3
beechwood smoked	●	0.5	–	49	8.5	1.5
Parma	●	0.1	–	120	12.5	7.5
Wiltshire	●	0.8	0.6	101	10	6.4
Yorkshire	●	0.2	0.3	70	10.5	3
Haslet, 50g	●	9.5	0.4	72	6.5	1
Kabanos, 50g	●	0.5	0.3	120	12	7.5
Liver pâté, 50g	●	0.4	n/a	174	6.3	16.4
reduced fat	●	1.5	Tr	96	9	6
Liver sausage, 50g	●	3	n/a	113	6.7	8.4
Luncheon meat, canned, 50g	●	1.8	n/a	140	6.5	11.9
Pâté, Brussels, 50g	●	2	0.1	173	6	15.5
Pepperami, hot, 50g	●	1.3	0.6	277	9.5	26
Pork salami sausage, 50g	●	0.9	0.1	268	11	24.5
Polony, 50g	●	7.1	n/a	141	4.7	10.6
Pork, 50g:						
luncheon meat	●	1.7	–	134	7	11
oven-baked	●	0.7	0.4	92	13	4
Salami, 50g:						
Danish	●	0.3	–	302	7.8	30

TIP: Poultry skin is high in calories – removing it from a chicken breast can cut calories by a third – and it is also high in saturated fats.

Food type	**GL**	**Carb (g)**	**Fibre (g)**	**Cal (kcal)**	**Pro (g)**	**Fat (g)**
Salami, *contd:*						
German	●	0.5	–	198	9.5	17.5
Milano	●	1.5	–	214	11.5	18
Scotch eggs, 100g	●	13.1	–	241	12	16
Tongue, lunch, 50g	●	0.2	–	88	9.8	5.2
Turkey, breast, roasted, 50g	●	0.3	–	58	12.5	0.7

TIP: Roast skinless chicken breasts quickly in an oven set to 200°C/gas mark 6. Warm a teaspoonful of olive oil in an ovenproof dish, rinse the chicken breasts and pat them dry, then roll them over in the warm oil. Sprinkle herbs on top and return the dish to the oven. Cook for 15 minutes, but check them halfway through and flip them over. Flip them back a few minutes later to brown the tops.

OILS AND FATS

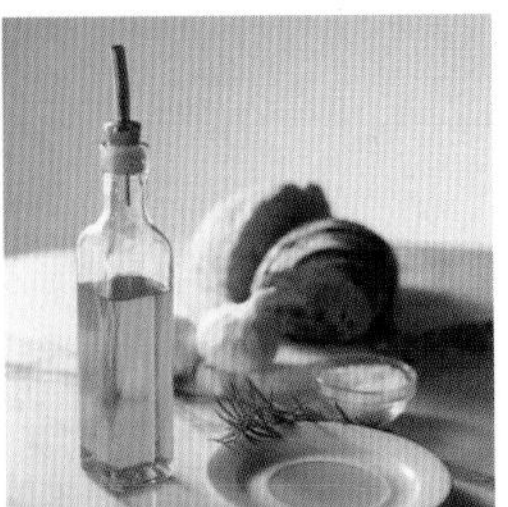

Though carb-free, oils and fats contain 9 calories of fat per gram, which can add up to a lot in total. Not all fats are the same in terms of their nutritional value. It's best to opt for those with the highest level of monounsaturated fats, like olive and rapeseed oils, or those high in omega-3 fatty acids. Avoid saturated fats as much as you can; that means restricting butter, lard, meat dripping, pork crackling, suet, coconut and palm oils. See pages 33-4 for more information on fats and oils.

TIP: Labels can be misleading. Rapeseed oil, which is good for you, may just be listed as 'vegetable oil' on the label. Meanwhile, 'blended' oils often contain palm oil, a saturated fat that has been treated during blending, and which is not good for you.

Food type	GL	Carb (g)	Fibre (g)	Cal (kcal)	Pro (g)	Fat (g)
Coconut oil, 1 tbsp		–	n/a	135	Tr	15
Cooking fat, 1 tbsp		–	–	135	–	15
Corn oil, 1 tbsp		–	–	124	–	13.8
Dripping, beef, 1 tbsp		Tr	–	134	Tr	14.9
Ghee:						
butter, 1 tbsp		Tr	n/a	135	Tr	15
palm, 1 tbsp		Tr	–	135	Tr	15
Lard, 1 tbsp		–	n/a	134	Tr	14.9
Olive oil, 1 tbsp		–	n/a	135	Tr	15
Palm oil, 1 tbsp		–	n/a	135	Tr	15
Peanut oil, 1 tbsp		–	n/a	135	Tr	15
Rapeseed oil, 1 tbsp		–	n/a	135	Tr	15
Safflower oil, 1 tbsp		–	n/a	135	Tr	15
Sesame oil, 1 tbsp		–	n/a	138	–	15.3
Soya oil, 1 tbsp		–	n/a	135	Tr	15
Stir-fry oil, 1 tbsp		0.1	Tr	122	–	13.5
Suet, shredded, 1 tbsp		1.8	n/a	124	Tr	13
Sunflower oil, 1 tbsp		–	–	124	–	13.8
Vegetable oil, 1 tbsp		–	–	135	Tr	15
Wheatgerm oil, 1 tbsp		–	–	135	Tr	15
For butter and margarine:						
see under Dairy						

TIP: Oil goes cloudy if it gets cold, but will return to normal once it warms up again. Don't keep oils too long as they can go off.

PASTA AND PIZZA

There is a considerable difference between the GI and GL values of pasta. Though most are low or medium GI they are almost all high GL, once portion size is taken into account. Keep pasta as an accompaniment rather than making it the focus of a meal. Though white and wholemeal pasta have similar GL ratings, wholemeal contains more fibre so is better for you. Pizza should be avoided completely during the weight-loss phase. Try not to buy ready-made pasta sauces as the sugar content is frequently sky high.

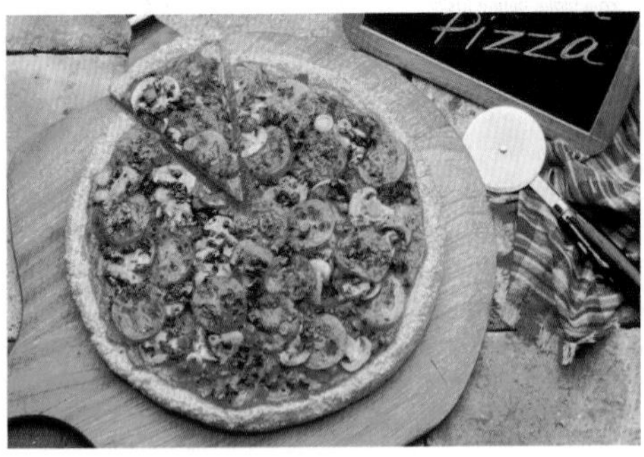

TIP: Avoid canned pasta. It usually contains large quantities of sugar and other undesirable ingredients like stabilisers and acidity regulators.

Food type	GL	Carb (g)	Fibre (g)	Cal (kcal)	Pro (g)	Fat (g)
Pasta						
Dried lasagne sheets, cooked weight 100g:						
standard	●	18.1	n/a	89	3.1	0.4
verdi	●	18.3	n/a	93	3.2	0.4
Dried pasta shapes, cooked weight 100g:						
standard	●	18.1	n/a	89	3.1	0.4
verdi	●	18.3	n/a	93	3.2	0.4
Fresh egg pasta, 100g:						
conchiglie, penne, fusilli	●	31	1.4	170	7	2
lasagne sheets	●	29	4.6	150	6	1.1
spaghetti	●	24	1	129	5	1.4
tagliatelle	●	24	1	129	5	1
Macaroni, boiled, 100g	●	18.5	n/a	86	3	0.5
Spaghetti, cooked weight 100g:						
dried, egg	●	22.2	n/a	104	3.6	0.7
wholemeal	●	23.2	n/a	113	4.7	0.9
Stuffed fresh pasta, 100g:						
four cheese tortellini	○	20.1	0.9	133	5.6	3.3
spinach & ricotta tortellini verdi	○	24	2.7	163	6	4.5

TIP: If you can't avoid pasta or pizza you can moderate their effects by choosing a healthy sauce such as fresh tomato, or selecting a plain, thin-based pizza and accompanying it with a green salad.

Food type	GL	Carb (g)	Fibre (g)	Cal (kcal)	Pro (g)	Fat (g)
Stuffed fresh pasta, *contd:*						
ham & cheese tortellini	●	13	1.7	170	6	6
cheese & porcini ravioli	●	21.6	2.8	164	7.8	5.2
Pasta Sauces						
Amatriciana, fresh, low fat, 100ml	●	5	1	155	4.4	13
Arrabbiata, fresh, low fat, 100ml	●	7	0.7	48	1.2	1.7
Bolognese, 100ml	●	2.5	n/a	161	11.8	11.6
Carbonara:						
fresh, 100ml	●	4.8	0.5	196	6	17
fresh, low fat, 100ml	●	5	0.5	81	5	4.5
Pesto:						
fresh, homemade, 100ml	●	6	1.4	45	2.2	1.3
green pesto, jar, 100ml	●	5	0.8	374	5	39
red pesto, jar, 100ml	●	3.1	0.4	358	4.1	36.6
Tomato & basil, fresh, 100ml	●	8.8	1.3	51	1.8	0.9
Canned Pasta						
Ravioli in tomato sauce, 200g can	●	26.4	0.6	146	6.2	1.6
Spaghetti bolognese, 200g can	●	26.4	1	158	6.8	3

TIP: Gluten-free corn and rice pastas still have a high GL value.

Food type	GL	Carb (g)	Fibre (g)	Cal (kcal)	Pro (g)	Fat (g)
Spaghetti hoops, 200g		22.2	1	106	3.4	0.4
Spaghetti in tomato sauce, 200g can		26	1	122	3.4	0.4
diet, 200g		20.2	1.2	100	3.6	0.4
Spaghetti with sausages in tomato sauce, 200g		21.6	1	176	7	6.8
Spicy pepperoni pasta, 200g can		18.2	1	166	5.8	7.8
Spicy salsa twists, 200g		21.8	1.6	150	5.4	4.6
Pasta Ready Meals						
Bolognese shells Italiana, *diet*, per 100g		9.6	0.8	71	5.2	1.3
Canneloni bolognese, per 100g		11.8	n/a	149	6.1	8.3
Deep pasta bake, chicken & tomato, per 100g		13	1.3	95	4.5	3
Lasagne, each		14.6	n/a	191	9.8	10.8
vegetable, per 100g		12.6	0.9	110	5.3	4.7
Pasta bolognese, per 100g		54	n/a	375	18	9.6
Ravioli bianche, 100g		29.7	n/a	200	9.6	4.7

TIP: Never overcook pasta; it just raises the GL further. Keep it al dente (with some bite to it) rather than letting it get very soft. Test a piece a few minutes before the recommended cooking time is up.

Food type	GL	Carb (g)	Fibre (g)	Cal (kcal)	Pro (g)	Fat (g)
Risotto, beef, per pack	●	57.8	5.6	346	15.3	5.9
Spaghetti bolognese, per pack	●	60	3.7	445	26	11
Pizza						
Cheese & onion deep filled pizza, 100g slice	●	30.3	1.3	223	8.4	8.2
Cheese & tomato pizza, 100g slice:	●	24.8	1.5	235	9	11.8
deep pan base	●	35.1	n/a	249	12.4	7.5
French bread base	●	31.4	–	230	10.6	7.8
thin base	●	33.9	n/a	277	14.4	10.3
French bread pizza, 100g slice	●	31	1.5	240	11	7.5
Ham & mushroom pizza, 100g slice	●	29.5	1.1	227	11.4	7.5
Pepperoni & sausage pizza, 100g slice	●	28.1	2.2	303	11.6	16
Pepperoni deep crust pizza, 100g slice	●	29.2	1.7	263	10.6	11.5
Pizza bases, 20cm diameter:						
deep pan	●	56	n/a	298	8.5	4.4
standard	●	56	n/a	298	8.5	4.4
stone baked	●	55	n/a	274	8.5	2.2

TIP: If you find one brand of wholemeal pasta stodgy, then try another; they have improved a lot recently.

Food type	GL	Carb (g)	Fibre (g)	Cal (kcal)	Pro (g)	Fat (g)
Pizza topping, 100g:						
spicy tomato	●	9	1	66	1.6	2.6
tomato, cheese, onion & herbs	●	8.1	0.9	80	3	4
tomato, herbs & spices	●	9.4	0.8	67	1.5	2.6
For more pizzas: *see under* Fast food						

TIP: Stuffed pasta may have a slightly lower GL than plain pasta, but it has a much higher fat content. Approach with caution.

PIES AND QUICHES

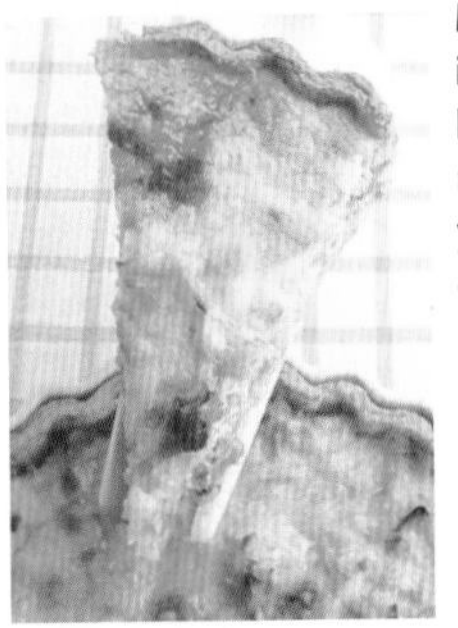

Most pastry is high GL, and is also high in fat while being low in fibre. If you must eat pies or quiches, you can minimise their effects by going for wholemeal pastry and low-GL fillings, limiting the portion size and accompanying it with a heap of salad leaves or lightly steamed green vegetables. Avoid any pies that are encased in pastry. Those with a potato topping – like a fish pie – are better than those with a pastry top but should still be avoided during the weight-loss phase of a GL diet.

TIP: Raw wholemeal pastry tends to crumble more easily than white, so be careful when lifting it. If you roll it on a board you can hold a flan tin over the board and turn the board over, instead of trying to manoeuvre the pastry itself.

Food type	GL	Carb (g)	Fibre (g)	Cal (kcal)	Pro (g)	Fat (g)
Chicken & mushroom pie, individual	●	25	1	321	8	21
Cornish pasty, each	●	25	n/a	267	6.7	16.3
Game pie, 100g	●	34.7	n/a	381	12.2	22.5
Pastry, 100g cooked:						
flaky	●	46	n/a	564	5.6	41
shortcrust	●	54.3	n/a	524	6.6	32.6
wholemeal	●	44.6	n/a	501	8.9	33.2
Pork pie, individual	●	23.7	n/a	363	10.8	25.7
Quiche Lorraine, 100g:	●	19.6	n/a	358	13.7	25.5
cheese & egg, white pastry	●	17.1	n/a	315	12.4	22.3
cheese & egg, wholemeal pastry	●	14.5	1.9	308	13.2	22.4
Sausage rolls, each:						
flaky pastry	●	25.4	n/a	383	9.9	27.6
short pastry	●	19.4	0.8	289	11.1	19.3
Shepherd's pie, diet 100g	○	10.1	0.9	73	3.5	2.1
Steak & kidney pie, canned, 100g	●	11.8	n/a	169	7.7	10.1
Yorkshire pudding, each	○	31	2.4	241	9	9

TIP: Make your own shepherd's pie, but keep it low fat and use mashed sweet potato for the topping instead of ordinary potatoes.

RICE AND NOODLES

Rice has either a medium or high GI, but once portion sizes are considered the GL is uniformly high. Don't choose it; go for extra vegetables instead. If this is impossible, then basmati, brown rice and wild rice (actually a grass seed) are the best choices. Never have more than 2 tablespoons of cooked rice. Easy-cook rice and glutinous rice, like that served in oriental restaurants, should always be avoided. Some noodles are medium GL, but again portion size is critical.

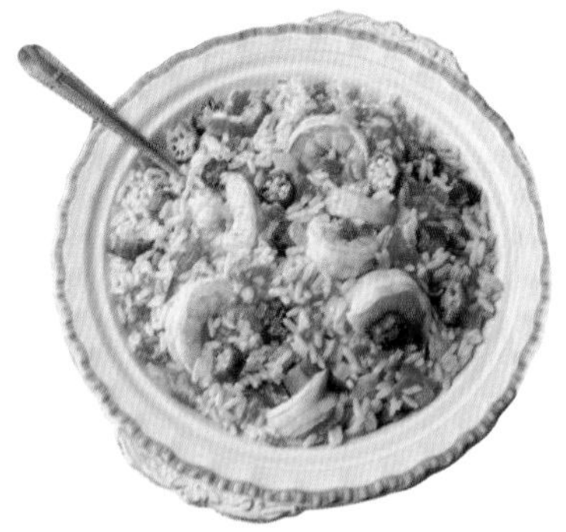

TIP: Wild rice has a good fibre content, and delicious flavour, but it is expensive. Mix it with basmati rice for an attractive dish.

Food type	GL	Carb (g)	Fibre (g)	Cal (kcal)	Pro (g)	Fat (g)
Rice, cooked						
Arborio rice, 75g	●	23.3	0.3	105	2.2	0.3
Basmati rice, 75g	●	22.4	n/a	113	2	1.7
Brown rice, 75g	●	24	0.6	106	2	0.6
Egg fried rice, 75g	●	19.3	0.3	156	3.2	8
Long grain rice, 75g	●	22.6	–	103	2.1	0.3
Long grain & wild rice, 75g	●	27.8	–	104	3.4	0.4
Pilau rice, 75g	●	23	0.5	106	2.7	0.4
Pudding rice, 75g	●	24.2	0.2	107	1.9	0.3
Risotto rice, 75g	●	23.3	0.3	105	2.2	0.3
Short grain rice, 75g	●	26	0.7	108	2	0.3
White rice:						
plain, 75g	●	23.2	0.1	104	2	1
easy cook, 75g	●	23.2	n/a	104	2	1
Wholegrain rice, 75g	●	21.2	0.6	102	2.7	0.7
Noodles, cooked						
Egg noodles, 75g	○	9.8	0.5	47	2	0.4
Stir fry noodles, 75g	●	23.8	1.1	107	2.2	0.4
Thai rice noodles, 75g	●	26	0.7	108	2	0.3
Thread noodles, 75g	○	7.4	–	51	1.8	1.5

TIP: You don't just need to watch the quantity of rice you eat; you also need to make sure it is not overcooked. Cooking breaks down the starches and can increase the GL, so keep it nutty.

SNACKS, NIBBLES AND DIPS

Snacks are an important part of a GL diet, preventing any blood-sugar dips between meals, but they do need to be the right ones. Nuts are frequently recommended: 10–15 almonds is about the right quantity, or about 30 pistachios. Olives are in many ways the ideal snack; they are comparatively low in fat and calories – especially if you buy olives in brine rather than oil – and have a low GL. As far as dips are concerned, the best option is often to make your own, controlling the ingredients. If you don't, then check labels carefully.

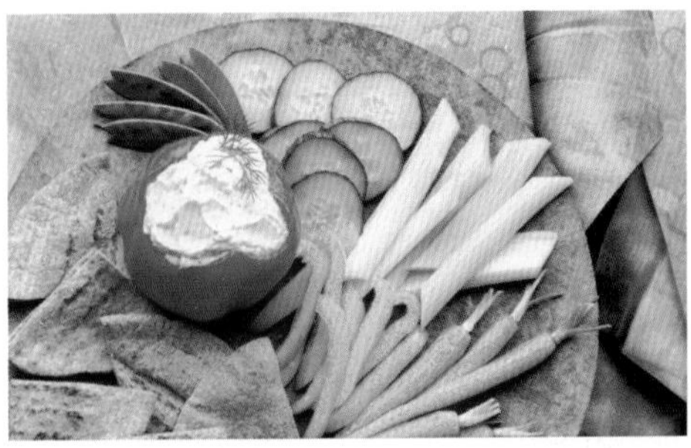

TIP: Nuts and seeds are high in fibre as well as protein, magnesium, folic acid and vitamin E.

Food type	GL	Carb (g)	Fibre (g)	Cal (kcal)	Pro (g)	Fat (g)
Crisps						
Cheese corn snacks, per pack (21g)	●	11.3	0.2	110	1.7	6.3
Hoop snacks, per pack (27g)	●	20.5	0.6	175	1.1	9.7
Potato crisps:						
cheese & onion, per pack (34.5g)	●	17.9	1.6	176	2.1	10.7
lightly salted, 25g	●	13.8	1.3	121	1.6	6.7
mature cheddar with chives, 25g	●	13.6	1.3	120	2	6.4
pickled onion, per pack (34.5g)	●	17.6	1.6	173	1.9	10.6
prawn cocktail, per pack (34.5g)	●	16.9	1.5	180	2	11.6
ready salted, per pack (34.5g)	●	17.8	1.6	179	1.9	11.1
roast chicken, (light), per pack (28g)	●	17.9	1.7	176	2.1	10.7
salsa with mesquite, 25g	●	13.8	1.4	116	1.5	6.1
salt & vinegar, per pack (34.5g)	●	17.7	1.5	173	1.8	10.6
salt & vinegar, (light), per pack (28g)	●	14.6	1.4	112	1.8	5

TIP: Don't forget to eat two snacks a day to keep your blood sugar levels steady; just make sure they're good for you. Take batons of carrot, apples and oatcakes to work. If there's nothing healthy to hand, you're more likely to be tempted by crisps or chocolate.

Food type	GL	Carb (g)	Fibre (g)	Cal (kcal)	Pro (g)	Fat (g)
Potato crisps, *contd:*						
sea salt with balsamic vinegar, 25g		13.4	1.2	122	1.7	6.9
smokey bacon, per pack (34.5g)		16.9	1.5	181	2	11.6
Quavers, per pack (20g)		12.2	0.2	103	0.6	5.8
Wheat crunchies:						
bacon flavour, per pack (35g)		19.6	1.4	172	3.4	8.9
salt & vinegar, per pack (35g)		19.1	0.9	170	3.7	8.7
spicy tomato, per pack (35g)		19.6	1.4	172	3.3	8.9
Worcester sauce, per pack (35g)		19.7	1.4	172	3.3	8.9
Nibbles						
Bombay mix, 50g		19.2	5.3	254	5.6	17.2
Breadsticks, each		3.6	0.2	21	0.6	0.4
Japanese rice crackers, 50g		39.5	0.3	200	4.7	2.6
Nachos, 100g		31	–	230	4	10
Olives, 15g black		3.4	1.7	32	0.2	1.0
Peanuts & raisins, 50g		15.9	2.4	237	8.8	15.3
yoghurt coated, 50g		27.2	1	233	4.5	12.9
Popcorn						
candied, 50g		38.8	n/a	240	1.1	10
plain, 50g		24.4	n/a	297	3.1	21.4

TIP: Watch plain popcorn. It has a low GL, so it's fine in moderation – but moderation is difficult and the calorie count is high.

Food type	GL	Carb (g)	Fibre (g)	Cal (kcal)	Pro (g)	Fat (g)
Poppadums, each:						
fried in veg oil	●	9.7	–	92	4.4	4.2
spicy, microwaved	●	10.7	3.2	64	5	0.1
Prawn crackers, 25g	●	10.3	0.3	77	0.2	3.9
Tortilla chips						
chilli flavour, 50g	●	31	n/a	248	3.5	13
cool original, per pack (40g)	●	25	1.4	204	3	10.5
jalapeño cheese flavour, 50g	●	30.5	n/a	260	3.5	13.5
pizza, per pack (40g)	●	23	1.4	202	3	11
salsa flavour, 50g	●	32.5	n/a	247	3.5	13
salted, 50g	●	30	2.5	230	3.8	11.3
tangy cheese, per pack (40g)	●	23	1.2	204	3.2	11
Trail mix, 50g	●	18.6	n/a	216	4.6	14.3
Twiglets, 50g	●	28.7	5.7	192	6.2	5.9
curry	●	28	3	225	4	10.7
tangy	●	28	2.8	227	4	2.8
Dried Fruit						
Apple rings, 25g	●	15	2.4	60	0.5	0.1
Apricots, 25g	●	9.1	n/a	40	1	0.2
Banana, 25g	●	13.4	2.4	55	0.8	0.2

TIP: Drain some black olives in brine and rinse well under running water; put them in a bowl, add some chopped fresh herbs and a drizzle of olive oil. Stir well and serve.

Food type	GL	Carb (g)	Fibre (g)	Cal (kcal)	Pro (g)	Fat (g)
Banana chips, 25g	●	16.2	2	133	0.4	7.4
Currants, 25g	●	17	n/a	67	0.6	0.1
Dates, flesh & skin, 25g	●	17	n/a	68	0.8	0.1
Figs, 25g	●	13.2	n/a	57	0.9	0.4
Fruit salad, 25g	●	11.1	1.8	46	0.8	0.2
Mixed fruit, 25g	●	17	n/a	67	0.6	0.1
Pineapple, diced, 25g	●	21	0.9	87	–	Tr
Prunes, 25g	●	9.6	1.6	40	0.7	0.1
Raisins, seedless, 25g	●	17.3	0.5	72	0.5	0.1
Sultanas, 25g	●	17.4	0.5	69	0.7	0.1
Nuts and Seeds						
Almonds:						
weighed with shells, 50g	●	1.3	1.4	115	3.9	10.3
flaked/ground, 25g	●	1.8	1.8	158	6.3	14
Brazils:						
weighed with shells, 50g	●	0.7	1.9	157	3.3	15.7
kernel only, 25g	●	0.8	1.3	170	3.5	17
Cashews:						
kernel only, 25g	●	4.5	0.8	144	4.5	12
pieces, 25g	●	4.3	0.8	156	6	12.7

TIP: Hummus makes a great dip, and is rich in B vitamins. Make your own, blending cooked chickpeas, some of their cooking liquid, tahini (sesame seed paste), lemon juice, garlic and a little olive oil.

Food type	GL	Carb (g)	Fibre (g)	Cal (kcal)	Pro (g)	Fat (g)
Chestnuts, kernel only, 25g	○	9.2	n/a	43	0.5	0.7
Coconut: *see under* Fruit						
Hazelnuts:						
weighed with shell, 50g	●	1.2	1.3	124	2.7	12.1
kernel only, 25g	●	1.5	1.5	167	4.3	16
Hickory nuts: *see* Pecans						
Macadamia nuts, salted, 50g	●	2.4	n/a	374	4	38.8
Mixed nuts, 25g	●	2	n/a	152	5.7	13.5
Monkey nuts: *see* Peanuts						
Peanuts:						
plain, weighed with shells, 50g	●	4.3	2.2	195	8.9	15.9
plain, kernel only, 25g	●	3.1	–	141	6.5	11.5
dry roasted, 50g	●	5.2	n/a	295	12.9	24.9
roasted & salted, 50g	●	3.6	n/a	301	12.4	26.5
Pecans, kernel only, 25g	●	1.5	1.2	175	2.8	17.5
Pine nuts, kernel only, 25g	●	1	n/a	172	3.5	17.2
Pistachios, weighed with	●					
shells, 50g	●	2.3	1.7	83	2.5	7.7
Poppy seeds, 10g	●	1.9	–	56	2.1	4.4
Pumpkin seeds, 25g	●	3.8	1.3	142	6.1	11.4
Sesame seeds, 10g	●	0.6	0.7	64	2.3	5.8
Sunflower seeds, 25g	●	4.7	1.5	145	5	11.9

TIP: Consider alternatives to nuts. Pumpkin seeds are rich in minerals and are delicious toasted in a dry frying pan, as are sunflower seeds.

Food type	GL	Carb (g)	Fibre (g)	Cal (kcal)	Pro (g)	Fat (g)
Walnuts:						
weighed with shell, 50g	●	0.7	0.8	148	3.2	14.7
halves , 25g	●	0.8	0.9	172	3.7	17.1
Dips						
Curry & mango dip, 100g	●	6.1	–	334	4.5	32.4
Mexican dips, 100g:						
guacamole	●	86	n/a	140	n/a	12.2
Mexican bean	●	12.1	2.4	89	2.7	3.3
spicy	●	4.8	–	324	4.7	31.7
Hummus, 100g	●	11.6	n/a	187	7.6	12.6
Onion & chive dip, 100g	●	5.6	0.5	283	4.6	26.9
Salsa, 100g						
cheese	●	9.3	n/a	143	2.5	10.7
cool, organic	●	6.3	1.2	141	1.1	0.4

TIP: Dips don't have to be accompanied by bread. Try tomato wedges, crisp lettuce leaves, fennel slices, celery sticks, strips of carrot, pepper and cucumber, hard-boiled eggs, little sausages, spring onions, radishes, button mushrooms and cauliflower florets. There are several dip recipes in this book, including tomato salsa (page 91), tuna dip (page 123), hummus (page 164) and aubergine dip (page 201). Make your own guacamole by mixing 2 mashed avocados, 2 tbsp lemon juice, a crushed clove of garlic, ½ chopped red onion, 2 chopped tomatoes, a finely chopped green chilli (if liked) and some fresh coriander.

Food type	GL	Carb (g)	Fibre (g)	Cal (kcal)	Pro (g)	Fat (g)
Salsa, *contd*:						
hot, organic	●	6.2	1.1	141	1.1	0.4
picante	●	4.6	–	28	1.4	0.5
Sour-cream based dips, 100g	●	4	n/a	360	2.9	37
Taramasalata, 100g	●	4.1	n/a	504	3.2	52.9
Tzatziki, 100g	●	1.9	n/a	66	3.8	4.9

TIP: Don't keep nuts too long as the oils they contain will go rancid. Buy little and often.

SOUP

Many soups are OK for the GL dieter, but by far the best bet is to make your own, as commercial brands often contain sugars and are thickened with flour, potato or gum. Soup is quickly and easily made at home and excess can be frozen for an almost-instant meal. Watch your use of root vegetables and don't be tempted to add ingredients like cream or pasta. Croûtons on top are not a good idea, and try to avoid accompanying soup with bread. Most of your existing soup recipes will easily adapt to GL eating.

TIP: Cold soups are refreshing. Blend 300g low-fat natural yoghurt with two chopped, deseeded tomatoes, a peeled and chopped small cucumber, a chopped clove of garlic, a handful of coriander leaves and half a pint of skimmed milk. Chill for at least 30 minutes, stir well, check the seasoning and garnish with some coriander leaves before serving.

Food type	GL	Carb (g)	Fibre (g)	Cal (kcal)	Pro (g)	Fat (g)
Canned Soups						
Beef broth, 200ml		13.8	2	86	4.4	1.4
Beef consommé, 200ml		1.4	–	26	5.2	Tr
Beef & vegetable soup, 200ml		14.4	2	96	5.8	1.6
Broccoli soup, 200ml		11.8	0.8	90	2.6	3.6
Broccoli & potato soup, 200ml		11.6	1.4	62	2.6	0.6
Carrot & butter bean soup, 200ml		154	3.4	108	3.2	3.8
Carrot & coriander soup, 200ml		12	1.6	82	1.6	3
Carrot & lentil soup, *low calorie*, 200ml		12	1.6	62	2.8	0.2
Carrot, parsnip & nutmeg organic, 200ml		11.4	2	54	1.4	0.4
Chicken broth, 200ml		10.8	1.2	68	3	0.8
Chicken soup, *low calorie*, 200ml		8.2	–	60	2.4	2
Chicken & ham, 200ml		13.8	1.4	92	4.3	2
low calorie		8.8	0.9	59	1.1	2.2
Chicken & sweetcorn soup, 200ml		12.4	1.2	78	3.2	1.8
Chicken & vegetable soup, 200ml		12.2	2.4	72	3.4	1

TIP: The liquid used for cooking lentils makes an excellent base for a strong-flavoured soup. Reserve it if it's not needed for the lentil dish itself.

Food type	GL	Carb (g)	Fibre (g)	Cal (kcal)	Pro (g)	Fat (g)
Chicken & white wine soup, 200ml		7.6	n/a	94	1.8	6.4
Chicken noodle soup, *low calorie,* 200ml		6.2	0.4	34	1.4	0.2
Cock-a-leekie soup, 200ml		8.2	0.6	46	1.8	0.6
Consommé, 200ml		1.2	n/a	16	3	–
Cream of asparagus, 200ml		12	0.4	134	2.2	8.6
Cream of celery soup, 200ml		6	n/a	92	1.2	7.2
Cream of chicken soup, 200ml		12.2	0.2	138	3.6	8.4
Cream of chicken & mushroom, 200ml		9.2	0.2	100	3.2	5.6
Cream of mushroom, 200ml		11	0.2	126	1.8	8.2
Cream of tomato, 200ml		13.2	0.8	114	1.8	6
Creamy chicken with vegetables, fresh soup, 200ml		11	0.8	194	3.8	15
Cullen skink, 200ml		15.4	0.8	172	12.8	6.6
French onion soup, 200ml		8.6	0.8	42	1.4	0.2
Garden pea & mint fresh soup, 200ml		12.2	3	124	4.6	6.4
Italian bean & pasta soup, 200ml		15.8	2.2	84	4	0.6
Lentil soup, 200ml		14.8	2	80	4.6	0.4

TIP: Don't use potatoes to thicken soup. Choose soups that don't need extra thickening, or use a rough purée of cooked haricot beans.

Food type	GL	Carb (g)	Fibre (g)	Cal (kcal)	Pro (g)	Fat (g)
Lobster bisque, 200ml		8.2	0.4	92	6	4
Mediterranean tomato, 200ml		13.6	1.4	66	2	0.4
Minestrone soup:						
chunky fresh, 200ml		11.8	1.8	68	2.6	1.2
Miso, 200ml		4.7	–	40	2.6	1.2
Mulligatawny beef curry soup 200ml		14.6	1.2	94	10.4	1.8
Mushroom soup:						
low calorie, 200ml		8.8	0.2	54	2	1.2
Oxtail soup, 200ml		13	0.6	74	3.2	1
Parsnip & carrot:						
low calorie, 200ml		10.6	1.8	50	1	0.4
Pea & ham, 200ml		16.6	2.4	110	6	2.2
Potato & leek, 200ml		16.2	1.6	90	2.2	1.8
Royal game, 200ml		12.4	0.4	82	5.6	1
Scotch broth, 200ml		15	1.8	94	3.8	2
Spicy parsnip, 200ml		12.2	3	102	2.2	5
Spicy tomato & rice with sweetcorn, 200ml		18.4	1	90	2.6	0.6
Spring vegetable soup, 200ml		12.4	1.4	62	1.6	0.8

TIP: Croûtons are not the only garnish for soup; try chopped basil over tomato soup or finely chopped cucumber over fennel soup. A few roughly chopped walnuts make a good croûton substitute when you want something crunchier. Slivers of chilli can be added to spicy soups.

Food type	GL	Carb (g)	Fibre (g)	Cal (kcal)	Pro (g)	Fat (g)
Thai chicken with noodles, 200ml		13.6	0.6	94	3.4	0.8
Tomato soup:						
low calorie, 200ml		9.4	0.6	52	1.4	1.0
Vegetable soup, 200ml		16.4	1.8	86	2	1.4
chunky fresh, 200ml		15.4	2.2	80	3.2	0.6
low calorie, 200ml		11.8	1.8	62	2	0.6
Winter vegetable soup, 200ml		16.4	2.2	92	5.6	0.4
low calorie, 200ml		12.0	1.6	62	3.2	0.2
Sachet/Cup Soups						
Beef & tomato cup soup, per sachet		15.8	1	83	1.4	1.6
Broccoli & cauliflower:						
thick & creamy, per sachet		13.7	2.7	107	1.6	5.1
low calorie, per sachet		10	0.5	59	0.9	1.7
Cajun spicy vegetable low calorie soup, per sachet		9.4	1.6	52	1.7	0.8
Cheese & broccoli cup soup, per sachet		23.5	1.9	160	5.2	5

TIP: If soup burns and sticks to the bottom of the pot, decant the unburnt ingredients carefully into a clean pan then check the taste. If it tastes burnt, you won't be able to rescue it and will have to start again. Otherwise, just carry on with the decanted soup.

Food type	GL	Carb (g)	Fibre (g)	Cal (kcal)	Pro (g)	Fat (g)
Chicken soup, cup soup						
per sachet		8.3	1.4	83	1.1	5
Chicken & leek cup soup,						
per sachet		12.2	1.7	96	1.2	4.7
Chicken & mushroom						
per sachet:		20.2	1.3	132	3.7	4
low calorie		9	0.9	60	1.3	2.1
Chicken & sweetcorn soup:						
low calorie, per sachet		8.5	0.9	55	1.2	1.8
Chicken noodle soup:						
per sachet		17	0.7	96	4.3	1.2
Chicken, noodle & vegetable:						
low calorie, per sachet		10	1.2	55	1.6	1
Chinese chicken cup soup						
per sachet		19.1	2	101	3.5	1.2
Cream of asparagus cup soup,						
per sachet		18	2.3	134	0.7	6.6
Cream of chicken & vegetable,						
cup soup, per sachet		18	2.2	137	1.3	6.6
Cream of mushroom, cup soup						
per sachet		15.2	2	121	0.9	6.3

TIP: Be very wary of adding salt to any stock or vegetable cooking water you are going to use for soup, as its flavour becomes intensified. Peppercorns make stock cloudy and impart a rather acrid, burnt taste.

Food type	GL	Carb (g)	Fibre (g)	Cal (kcal)	Pro (g)	Fat (g)
Cream of vegetable cup soup, per sachet	●	17.3	2.8	135	1.8	6.5
Creamy potato & leek cup soup, per sachet	●	15.5	3	109	1.9	4.4
Golden vegetable:						
cup soup, per sachet	○	14.3	0.9	83	1.1	2.4
low calorie, per sachet	●	9.7	1.5	58	1.1	1.7
Hot & sour cup soup, sachet	○	18.7	1.2	91	2.5	0.7
Leek & potato low calorie, per sachet	●	10.2	0.5	57	0.9	1.4
Mediterranean tomato: *low calorie* per sachet	●	9.6	0.7	58	1.1	1.7
Minestrone soup:						
cup soup, per sachet	●	16.5	1.2	98	1.6	2.8
low calorie, per sachet	●	9.9	1.3	56	1.3	1.2
Oxtail soup, per sachet	●	11.2	0.8	83	2.2	3.3

TIP: Make a tasty Italian lentil soup. Rinse 200g green lentils. Put them in enough water to cover, bring to the boil and simmer for 10 minutes; clear any froth that rises. In another pan cook a chopped onion and clove of garlic in a little olive oil. Add the contents of a large tin of chopped tomatoes and cook for a couple of minutes, then add a bay leaf and some dried mixed herbs. Drain the lentils and add to the tomatoes; add about a litre of fresh water. Cook until the lentils are soft, maybe 30 minutes. Check the seasoning and serve immediately.

Food type	GL	Carb (g)	Fibre (g)	Cal (kcal)	Pro (g)	Fat (g)
Spicy vegetable cup soup, per sachet	●	22.3	1.2	109	2.9	1
Tomato cup soup, per sachet	●	17.2	0.7	92	0.7	2.3
Tomato & vegetable cup soup, per sachet	●	18.4	2.1	108	2.8	2.6

TIP: Make a vegetable soup using tinned, drained and rinsed haricot beans, French beans, finely sliced leeks, and a couple of skinned and deseeded tomatoes. Cover these with water and cook them at a simmer until they are tender. Just before serving stir a tablespoon of pesto – the best you can find, but check the ingredients as some contain potato starch and sugar – into the hot soup.

SUGAR AND SWEETENERS

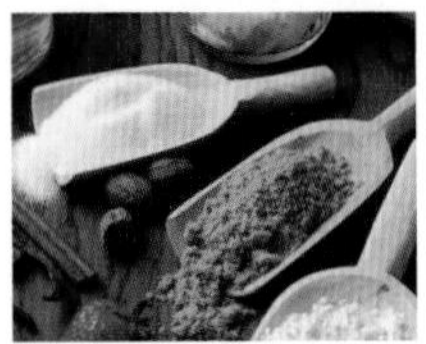

Using a little sugar is permissible on the GL diet, but a lot of packaged food already contains sugar and it is easy to push overall consumption up without realising it. Not all sugar is the same when it comes to GL; glucose and maltose have a higher GL than fructose, for example. Savoury foods may also contain sugar, as can low-fat products. Some sugar substitutes can have alarming effects on your digestion when consumed in even small quantities. Most dietitians suggest weaning yourself off sugar and sugar substitutes completely.

TIP: Remember that sugar can be found in all sorts of products, and can be described in many different ways on labels. Look out for dextrose, maltose, corn syrup, malto-dextrin, levulose, invert sugar, glucose syrup – all forms of sugar.

Food type	GL	Carb (g)	Fibre (g)	Cal (kcal)	Pro (g)	Fat (g)
Amber sugar crystals, 1 tsp	●	5	–	20	Tr	–
Date syrup, 1 tsp	●	3.7	Tr	15	0.1	–
Golden syrup, 1 tsp	●	4	–	15	–	–
Honey, 1 tsp	●	6.5	–	26	–	Tr
Icing sugar, 1 tsp	●	5	–	20	–	–
Jaggery	●	4.8	n/a	18	–	–
Maple syrup, 1 tsp	●	4.2	Tr	17	Tr	–
Molasses, 1 tsp	●	4	–	16	–	–
Sugar:						
caster, 1 tsp	●	5	–	20	–	–
dark brown, soft, 1 tsp	●	4.8	–	19	–	–
demerara, cane, 1 tsp	●	5	Tr	20	Tr	–
granulated, 1 tsp	●	5	–	20	–	–
light brown, soft, 1 tsp	●	4.7	–	19	–	–
preserving, 1 tsp	●	5	–	20	–	–
cube, white, each	●	5	–	20	–	–
Treacle, black, 1 tsp	●	3.3	n/a	13	0.1	–
Sweeteners						
Canderel, 1 tsp	●	0.47	–	1.9	0.01	–
Hermesetas, 1 tsp	●	0.28	0.21	1.4	0.01	–
Splenda, 1 tsp	●	0.5	–	2	–	–

TIP: If you can't live without sweetness, try granulated fructose or stevia, natural sweeteners that can be found in health-food shops.

SWEETS AND CHOCOLATES

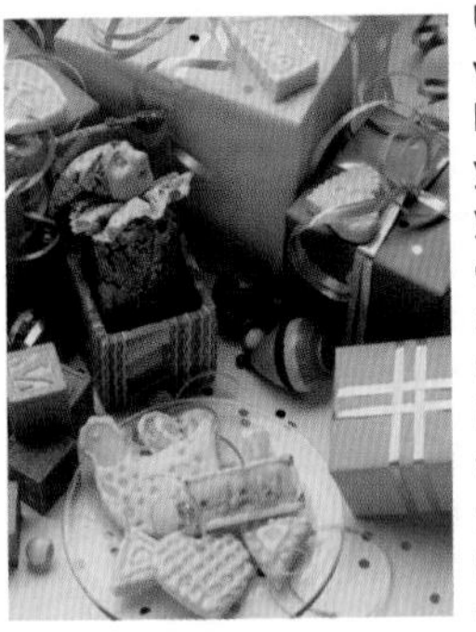

Unsurprisingly, there are virtually no green GL levels in this section. If you can do without, you'll find that sweet cravings disappear more quickly than you might expect; as Patrick Holford points out, your taste buds adapt relatively quickly. Fruit is a good substitute when you want something sweet, and a handful of grapes or berries, or a ripe plum, is much more satisfying than the instant glucose hit followed by an equally swift drop that your favourite sweets provide. Chocolate with a high cocoa content has lower levels of saturated fat and sugar, so you could allow yourself a little (not more than 20g) as a treat.

TIP: Chocolate and sweets are addictive. Always think before you buy, and try to refuse any that are offered. Chocolate-covered nuts are the best bet if you can't summon the willpower to say no completely.

Food type	**GL**	**Carb (g)**	**Fibre (g)**	**Cal (kcal)**	**Pro (g)**	**Fat (g)**
After Dinner Mints:						
dark chocolate, 25g	○	18.2	0.3	104	0.6	3.2
white chocolate, 25g	○	19.2	n/a	106	0.7	2.9
American Hard Gums, 25g	●	20.5	–	83	–	–
Barley Sugar, 25g	●	24.3	–	97.3	–	–
Black Jack chews, 25g	●	21.3	n/a	100	0.3	1.5
Blue Riband, 25g	●	16.6	0.3	128	1.2	6.3
Bonbons, 25g:						
buttermints	●	21.5	n/a	106	0.2	2.2
lemon	●	21	n/a	106	–	2.5
strawberry	●	19	n/a	95	–	2.3
toffee	●	21	n/a	105	–	2.3
Bounty, 25g:						
dark chocolate	●	14.4	n/a	120	0.8	0.6
milk chocolate	●	14.1	1.3	118	0.9	6.4
Breakaway, 25g	●	14.9	0.6	124	1.7	6.4
Buttermints, 25g	●	22.2	–	101	–	0.9
Butterscotch, 25g	●	22.5	–	103	–	1.4
Chocolate buttons, 25g	●	14	n/a	131	2	7.5
Caramel chocolate bar, 25g	○	13.6	–	141	1.5	9
Caramels, milk & plain chocolate, 25g	●	24.1	–	123	–	–

TIP: Note the portion sizes in the listings here if you feel tempted – 25g is the smallest bar of chocolate you can buy.

Food type	GL	Carb (g)	Fibre (g)	Cal (kcal)	Pro (g)	Fat (g)
Chewing gum:						
Airwaves, sugarfree , 5g		n/a	–	8	–	–
Doublemint, 5g		n/a	–	15	–	–
Extra peppermint, 5g		–	–	8	–	–
Ice White, sugarfree, 5g		–	–	9	–	–
Juicy Fruit, 5g		–	–	15	–	–
Peppermint, sugarfree, 5g		–	–	9	–	–
Spearmint, sugarfree, 5g		–	–	9	–	–
Chocolate cream, 25g	●	17.5	n/a	104	0.8	3.5
Chocolate éclairs, 25g	●	17.5	n/a	114	1	4.5
Chocolate limes, 25g	●	22.7	0.1	102	0.2	4.7
Chocolate Orange, 25g:						
dark chocolate	●	14.2	1.6	128	1	7.3
milk chocolate	●	14.5	0.5	133	1.9	7.4
Chocolate Truffles, 25g:						
with coffee liqueur	●	16	0.2	119	0.9	5.5
with orange liqueur	●	16	0.2	119	0.9	5.5
with whiskey cream	●	16	0.2	119	1	5.5
Chocolate, 25g:						
milk	○	14.2	n/a	130	1.9	7.7
plain	○	15.9	n/a	128	1.3	7

TIP: Read the ingredients on a popular chocolate bar and think about the health implications of the ones you recognise. That – and all the ones you don't know about – should make it easier to put back on the shelf.

Food type	GL	Carb (g)	Fibre (g)	Cal (kcal)	Pro (g)	Fat (g)
Chocolate, *contd*:						
white		14.6	n/a	132	2	7.7
raisin & biscuit		15.1	n/a	122	1.5	6.2
fruit & nut		13.8	n/a	123	2	6.5
wholenut		12	n/a	136	2.3	8.8
Coolmints, 25g		24.7	–	59	–	–
Cough candy, 25g		23.8	–	95.8	–	–
Cream toffees, assorted, 25g		18.3	–	108	0.9	3.5
Cream eggs, 25g		17.8	n/a	111	0.8	4
Crunchie, 25g		18	n/a	118	1	4.5
Dairy toffee, 25g		18.8	–	118	0.5	4.6
Double Decker, 25g		16.3	n/a	116	1.3	5.3
Energy Tablets, 25g						
glucose		22.3	n/a	90	Tr	–
orange		22.3	n/a	90	Tr	–
lemon		22.2	n/a	90	–	–
Everton mints, 25g		23.3	n/a	98	–	0.5
Flake bar, 25g		13.8	n/a	131	2	7.8
Fruit gums, 25g		19.3	n/a	84	1.5	–
Fruit pastilles, 25g		20.9	–	88	1.1	–
Fudge, 25g		18.3	n/a	109	0.8	3.8

TIP: Eat high-quality dark chocolate slowly. Let it dissolve in your mouth nibble by nibble, the way connoisseurs do, and really concentrate on the flavours. Good chocolate has a complex taste, so make the most of it.

Food type	GL	Carb (g)	Fibre (g)	Cal (kcal)	Pro (g)	Fat (g)
Galaxy (Mars), 25g:						
chocolate		14.2	–	133	2.3	7.5
caramel		15	–	122	1.3	6.3
double nut & raisin		13.9	–	134	13.9	7.7
hazelnut		12.1	–	143	1.9	9.7
praline		13	–	145	1.3	9.9
Jellies, assorted, 25g		23.5	n/a	95	–	–
Kit Kat, 25g:						
4-finger		15.4	0.3	127	1.5	6.6
Chunky		15.2	0.3	130	1.4	7
Lion Bar, 25g		16.9	0.2	122	1.2	5.6
Liquorice Allsorts, 25g		19	n/a	88	0.5	1.3
Lockets, 25g		24	n/a	96	–	–
M & Ms, 25g:						
chocolate		17.4	0.7	123	1.3	5.4
peanut		14.6	0.5	130	2.6	6.8
Maltesers, 25g		14.7	0.3	121	2.2	6
Mars Bar, 25g		17.3	0.3	112	1.1	4.4
Minstrels, 25g		17.8	n/a	127	1.3	5.6
Milky Way, 25g		18.7	0.4	110	0.9	3.5
Mint Crisp, 25g		16.4	1	121	0.9	5.8
Mint humbugs, 25g		22.4	–	103	0.2	1.5

TIP: Partly dip strawberries and cherries in melted dark chocolate; let them cool and serve beautifully arranged, garnished with mint.

Food type	GL	Carb (g)	Fibre (g)	Cal (kcal)	Pro (g)	Fat (g)
Mint imperials, 25g	●	24.5	n/a	99	–	–
Munchies, 25g:						
original	●	158	0.1	122	1.3	6
mint	●	16.9	0.4	108	1	4.1
Murray Mints, 25g	●	22.5	n/a	103	–	1.3
Orange Cream, 25g	●	18	n/a	105	0.8	3.5
Peanut Lion Bar, 25g	●	14.2	n/a	131	1.8	7.4
Pear Drops, 25g	●	24	n/a	96	–	–
Peppermints, 25g	●	25.7	n/a	98	0.1	0.2
Peppermint Cream, 25g	●	18.3	n/a	106	0.8	3.5
Picnic, 25g	●	14.8	n/a	118	1.8	5.8
Pineapple chunks, 25g	●	21	0.9	87	–	Tr
Polos:						
mints, 25g	●	24.6	–	101	–	0.3
sugar-free , 25g	●	24.8	–	60	–	–
smoothies, 25g	●	22.1	–	103	–	1.7
Pontefract cakes, 25g	●	16.7	0.6	70	0.6	0.1
Poppets, 25g:						
peanut	●	9.3	n/a	136	4.1	9.3
raisins	●	16.5	n/a	102	1.2	3.5
Refreshers, 25g	●	22.5	n/a	94	–	–
Revels, 25g	●	16.5	n/a	119	1.3	5.2

TIP: Choose chocolate with a high cocoa content (over 70%), even for cooking: it tastes much stronger, so you won't need as much.

Food type	GL	Carb (g)	Fibre (g)	Cal (kcal)	Pro (g)	Fat (g)
Ripple, 25g	●	14.8	n/a	132	1.7	7.3
Rolo, 25g	●	17.1	0.1	118	0.8	5.1
Sherbet Lemons, 25g	●	23.5	–	96	–	–
Snickers, 25g	○	8.8	0.3	70	1	3.5
Softfruits, 25g	●	23.8	n/a	95	–	0.3
Softmints, 25g	●	22	–	94	–	0.6
Spearmints, Extra Strong, 25g	●	24.8	n/a	99	–	–
Sugared almonds, 25g	○	19.5	0.6			
Sweet peanuts, 25g	○	20	0.4	107	0.8	0.4
Sweets, boiled, 25g	●	21.8	n/a	82	Tr	Tr
Toblerone, 25g	○	14.5	0.7	133	1.4	7.6
Toffees, mixed, 25g	●	16.7	n/a	107	0.6	4.7
Toffee Crisp, 25g	●	15.2	0.2	128	1.1	7
Toffo, 25g	●	17.5	–	113	0.5	4.5
Topic, 25g	●	15.1	0.4	126	1.6	6.6
Tunes, 25g	●	24.5	n/a	98	–	–
Turkish Delight, 25g	●	18.3	n/a	91	0.5	1.8
Twix, 25g	●	15.9	0.4	123	1.2	6.1

TIP: Be careful with sugar-free mints and chewing gums. The sugar substitute may be aspartame, about which some scientists have expressed serious reservations, or phenyl-alanine, which can act like a potent laxative. Other artificial sweeteners to watch out for include Acesulfame-K (E950), alitame, neotame, Neohesperidine DC (E959), Thaumatin (E957) and Xylitol (E967). Off-putting names, aren't they?

Food type	GL	Carb (g)	Fibre (g)	Cal (kcal)	Pro (g)	Fat (g)
Walnut whip, vanilla, 25g	●	15.2	0.2	124	1.5	6.4
Wine gums 25g	●	19.2	n/a	83	1.5	Tr

TIP: If you have a sweet habit do try to break it – it should only take about three weeks. The good news is that it takes about the same length of time to establish a new habit, like snacking on an apple, instead.

VEGETABLES

Almost all vegetables are low GL, apart from a few like potatoes, parsnips and sweet potatoes. Buy fresh or frozen rather than canned. Organic is preferable because they're free of pesticide residues and usually taste better. Don't overcook vegetables and save the cooking liquid for use as vegetable stock.

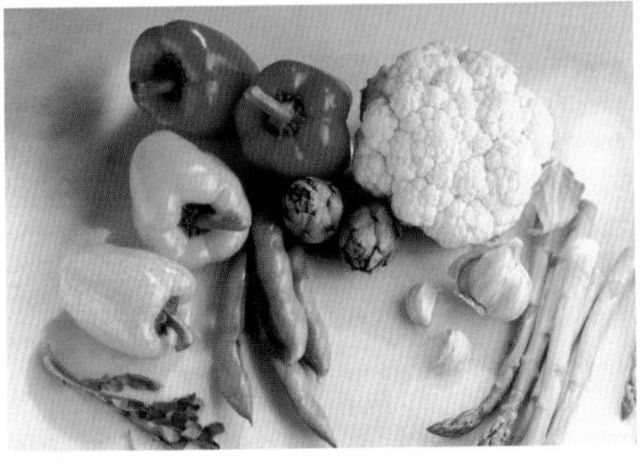

TIP: Make a simple fresh tomato sauce when tomatoes are cheap. Fry a chopped onion in a little olive oil, then add about 900g chopped tomatoes. Cook until soft, then purée in a blender; check for seasoning and if you are going to freeze it, don't season it at all. There are many variations; cook it with garlic, add herbs like thyme and basil. A green chilli, deseeded and chopped, will give it a kick.

Food type	GL	Carb (g)	Fibre (g)	Cal (kcal)	Pro (g)	Fat (g)
Artichokes, 1 globe	●	2.7	–	18	2.8	0.2
Artichoke, Jerusalem, boiled, 90g	●	9.5	–	37	1.4	0.1
Asparagus, 6 spears, boiled	●	1.1	n/a	21	2.7	0.6
Aubergine, half medium, fried	●	1.4	n/a	151	0.6	16
Avocado, half	●	1.6	n/a	160	1.6	16.4
Bamboo shoots, raw, 75g	●	0.8	0.2	5	0.5	0.1
Beans, broad, boiled, 75g	●	8.8	n/a	61	5.9	0.5
Beans, French, 100g boiled	●	4.7	n/a	25	1.7	0.1
Beans, runner, 50g, trimmed, boiled	●	1.2	n/a	9	0.6	0.3
Beansprouts, mung, 25g:						
raw	●	1	n/a	8	0.7	0.1
stirfried in blended oil	●	0.6	n/a	18	0.5	1.5
Beetroot, 90g:						
pickled	●	23.4	n/a	98	0.9	0.1
boiled	●	8.6	n/a	41	2.1	0.1
Broccoli, florets, boiled, 60g	●	0.7	n/a	14	1.9	0.5
Brussels sprouts, 6 trimmed, boiled	●	4.9	n/a	49	4.1	1.8

TIP: Cos lettuce keeps well in the fridge, has an excellent flavour and the smaller leaves make efficient and tasty scoops for dips. Always wash the leaves and dry them in a salad spinner or tea towel.

Food type	GL	Carb (g)	Fibre (g)	Cal (kcal)	Pro (g)	Fat (g)
Cabbage (Savoy, Summer), 75g:						
trimmed	●	3.1	n/a	20	1.3	0.3
shredded & boiled	●	1.7	n/a	12	0.8	0.3
Spring greens, raw	●	2.3	n/a	25	2.3	0.8
Spring greens, boiled	●	1.2	n/a	15	1.4	0.5
white	●	3.7	1.6	20	1.0	0.2
Carrot:						
1 medium, raw	●	7.9	n/a	35	0.6	0.3
1 medium, raw (young)	●	6.8	n/a	34	0.8	0.6
grated, 40g	●	3.2	1	15	0.2	0.1
boiled (frozen), 80g	●	3.8	1.8	18	0.3	0.2
boiled (young), 80g	●	3.5	n/a	18	0.5	0.3
Cassava, 100g:						
baked	●	40.1	1.7	155	0.7	0.2
boiled	●	33.5	1.4	130	0.5	0.2
Cauliflower, 100g:						
raw	●	3.0	n/a	34	3.6	0.9
boiled	●	2.1	n/a	28	2.9	0.9
Celeriac, 100g:						
flesh only, raw	●	5	0.4	29	1.3	0.4
flesh only, boiled	●	1.9	3.2	15	0.9	0.5

TIP: Sweet potatoes, the roots of a tropical vine, have a lower GL than true potatoes. Bake them in foil in a medium oven until they are soft. When the foil parcel gives to the touch, they are ready.

Food type	GL	Carb (g)	Fibre (g)	Cal (kcal)	Pro (g)	Fat (g)
Celery, 100g:						
stem only, raw		0.9	n/a	7	0.5	0.2
stem only, boiled		0.8	n/a	8	0.5	0.3
Chicory, 100g		2.8	n/a	11	0.5	0.6
Corn-on-the-cob						
boiled, 1 medium cob		13.3	n/a	76	2.9	1.6
mini corncobs, boiled, 100g		2.7	2.0	24	2.5	0.4
See also: Sweetcorn						
Courgettes (zucchini):						
trimmed, 50g		0.9	n/a	9	0.9	0.2
trimmed, boiled, 75g		1.5	n/a	14	1.5	0.3
trimmed, baked, 75g		1	n/a	16	1.1	0.2
fried in corn oil, 75g		2	n/a	47	2	3.6
Cucumber, trimmed, 75g		1.1	n/a	8	0.5	0.1
Eggplant: *see* Aubergine						
Fennel, Florence						
boiled, 75g		1.1	n/a	8	0.7	0.2
Garlic, half tsp purée or 1 clove, crushed		1.8	0.9	60	0.4	5.7
Gherkins,						
pickled, 75g		2	n/a	11	0.7	0.1
Ginger root, half tsp, grated	1	0.1	–	–	–	–

TIP: Try not to peel vegetables; removing the peel reduces the fibre content and also removes nutrients just below the skin.

Food type	GL	Carb (g)	Fibre (g)	Cal (kcal)	Pro (g)	Fat (g)
Greens, spring: *see* Cabbage						
Gumbo: *see* Okra						
Kale, curly, 40g:						
raw	●	0.6	n/a	13	1.4	0.6
shredded, boiled	●	0.4	n/a	10	1	0.4
Kohlrabi, 85g:						
raw	●	3.1	1.9	20	1.4	0.2
boiled	●	2.6	1.6	15	1.0	0.2
Ladies' Fingers: *see* Okra						
Leeks:						
trimmed, 60g	●	1.7	n/a	13	1.0	0.3
chopped, boiled, 100g	●	2.6	n/a	21	1.2	0.7
Lettuce, 1 cup (30g):						
green	●	0.5	n/a	4	0.2	0.2
iceberg	●	0.6	n/a	4	0.2	0.1
mixed leaf	●	0.9	0.8	5	0.3	–
Mediterranean salad leaves	●	0.9	0.5	6	0.3	0.1
spinach, rocket & watercress	●	0.4	0.4	7.5	0.9	0.3
Mange-tout, 50g:						
raw	●	2.1	n/a	16	1.8	0.1
boiled	●	1.7	n/a	13	1.6	0.1
stir-fried	●	1.8	n/a	36	1.9	2.4

TIP: When cooking red cabbage, add a little vinegar to the water to stop it from turning purple.

Food type	GL	Carb (g)	Fibre (g)	Cal (kcal)	Pro (g)	Fat (g)
Marrow:						
flesh only, 50g	●	1.1	n/a	6	0.3	0.1
flesh only, boiled, 75g	●	1.2	n/a	7	0.3	0.2
Mooli: *see* Radish, white						
Mushrooms, common, 40g:						
raw	●	0.2	n/a	5	0.7	0.2
boiled	●	0.2	0.4	4	0.7	0.1
fried in oil	●	0.1	n/a	63	1	6.5
canned	●	Tr	0.5	5	0.8	0.2
Mushrooms, oyster, 30g	●	–	0.1	2	0.5	0.1
Mushrooms, shiitake:						
boiled, 40g	●	4.9	–	22	0.6	0.1
dried, 20g	●	12.8	–	59	1.9	0.2
Neeps (Scotland): *see* Swede						
Okra (gumbo, ladies' fingers):						
raw, 25g	●	2	–	10	0.5	–
boiled, 30g	●	0.8	n/a	8	0.8	0.3
stir-fried, 30g	●	1.3	n/a	81	1.3	7.8
Onions:						
raw, flesh only, 30g	●	2.4	n/a	11	0.4	0.1
boiled, 40g	●	1.5	0.3	7	0.2	–
cocktail, drained, 40g	●	1.2	n/a	6	0.2	–

TIP: Toss fresh baby spinach leaves in a little gently warmed olive oil and sprinkle dry-fried pine nuts and chopped almonds over the top.

Food type	GL	Carb (g)	Fibre (g)	Cal (kcal)	Pro (g)	Fat (g)
Onions, *contd*:						
fried in vegetable oil, 40g	●	5.6	n/a	66	0.9	4.5
pickled, drained, 40g	●	2.0	n/a	10	0.4	0.1
Parsnips, trimmed, peeled, boiled, 80g	●	10.3	n/a	53	1.3	1.0
Peas:						
no pod, 75g	●	8.5	n/a	62	5.1	1.1
boiled, 90g	●	9.0	n/a	71	6.0	1.4
canned, 90g	●	12.2	n/a	72	4.8	0.8
Peas, mushy, canned, 100g	●	13.8	n/a	81	5.8	0.7
Peas, processed, canned, 100g	●	17.5	n/a	99	6.9	0.7
See also: Petit pois						
See also under: Beans, Pulses and Cereals						
Peppers:						
green, raw, 40g	●	1.0	n/a	6	0.3	0.1
green, boiled, 50g	●	1.3	n/a	9	0.5	0.2
red, raw, 40g	●	2.6	n/a	13	0.4	0.2
red, boiled, 50g	●	3.5	n/a	17	0.6	0.2
yellow, raw, 40g	●	2.1	0.7	10	0.5	0.1
chilli, 15g	●	0.1	n/a	3	0.4	0.1

TIP: Grate celeriac into fine strips, cook it briefly in boiling water then chill it in cold water. Serve with a dressing made from low-fat crème fraîche with a little Dijon mustard mixed in.

Food type	GL	Carb (g)	Fibre (g)	Cal (kcal)	Pro (g)	Fat (g)
Peppers, *contd:*						
jalapeños, 15g	●	0.5	n/a	3.3	0.2	0.1
Petit pois:						
fresh, 75g	●	13.1	3.1	75	5.2	0.6
frozen, boiled, 100g	●	5.5	n/a	49	5	0.9
Potatoes, Chips and Fries						
Chips, 150g:						
crinkle cut, frozen, fried	●	50.1	n/a	435	5.4	25
French fries, retail	●	51	n/a	420	5	23.3
homemade, fried	●	45.2	n/a	284	5.9	10.1
microwave chips	●	48.2	n/a	332	5.4	14.4
oven chips	●	44.7	n/a	243	4.8	6.3
straight cut, frozen, fried	●	54	n/a	410	6.2	20.3
Croquettes, fried in oil, 100g	●	21.6	n/a	214	3.7	13.1
Hash browns, 100g	●	26.8	n/a	153	2.9	5
Mashed potato, instant, 125g:						
made with semi-skimmed milk	●	18.5	1.3	88	3	1.5
made with skimmed milk	●	18.5	1.3	83	3	0.1
made with water	●	16.9	n/a	71	1.9	0.1
made up with whole milk	●	18.5	1.2	95	3	1.5
Potato fritters, 100g	●	16.3	1.2	145	2	8
Potato waffles, 100g	●	30.3	n/a	200	3.2	8.2

TIP: Blanch raw onion in boiling water if it's too strong for you.

Food type	GL	Carb (g)	Fibre (g)	Cal (kcal)	Pro (g)	Fat (g)
Potatoes, new, 100g:						
boiled, peeled		17.8	n/a	75	1.5	0.3
boiled in skins		15.4	n/a	66	1.4	0.3
canned		15.1	n/a	63	1.5	0.1
Potatoes, old, 90g:						
baked, flesh & skin		28.5	n/a	122	3.5	0.2
baked, flesh only		16.2	n/a	69	2.0	0.1
boiled, peeled		15.3	n/a	65	1.6	0.1
mashed with butter & milk		14	n/a	94	1.6	3.9
roast in oil/lard		23.3	n/a	134	2.6	4.0
Pumpkin, flesh only, boiled, 75g		1.7	n/a	10	0.5	0.2
Radicchio, 30g		0.5	0.5	4	0.4	0.1
Radish, red, 6		1.1	n/a	7	0.4	0.1
Radish, white/mooli, 20g		0.6	–	3	0.2	–
Ratatouille, canned, 115g		8.1	1.2	58	1.2	2.3
Salsify:						
flesh only, raw, 40g		4.1	1.3	11	0.5	0.1
flesh only, boiled, 50g		4.3	1.8	12	0.6	0.2
Shallots, 30g		1.0	n/a	6	0.5	0.1
Spinach:						
raw, one cup, 30g		0.5	n/a	8	0.8	0.2
boiled, 90g		0.7	n/a	17	2.0	0.7
frozen, boiled, 90g		0.5	n/a	19	2.8	0.7
Spring onions, bulbs & tops, 30g		0.9	n/a	7	0.6	0.2

Food type	GL	Carb (g)	Fibre (g)	Cal (kcal)	Pro (g)	Fat (g)
Sprouts: *see* Brussels Sprouts						
Squash:						
flesh only, 50g	●	1.1	n/a	6	0.3	0.1
flesh only, boiled, 75g	●	1.2	n/a	7	0.3	0.2
Swede, flesh only, boiled, 90g	●	2.1	n/a	10	0.3	0.1
Sweet potato, boiled, 90g	●	18.5	n/a	76	1.0	0.3
Sweetcorn, kernels, 80g:						
canned, drained, re-heated	●	21.3	n/a	98	2.3	1.0
canned, no salt, no sugar	●	13.4	2	62	2.1	–
Tomatoes:						
1 medium	●	4.7	0.6	29	1.1	0.6
canned, whole, 100g	●	3	n/a	16	1	0.1
cherry, 6	●	5.3	1.7	31	1.2	0.5
1 medium, fried in oil	●	7.5	n/a	137	1.1	11.6
sun-dried, 30g	●	3.3	2	63	1.3	4.9
paste, 2 tbsp	●	5	n/a	27	1.7	0.1
passata, 200g	●	9	0.4	50	2.8	0.2
chopped, canned, 200g	●	7	n/a	44	2.2	0.8
Turnip, flesh only, boiled, 60g	●	1.2	n/a	7	0.4	0.1
Water chestnuts, canned, 40g	●	1.9	1	11	0.7	0.1
Yam, flesh only, boiled, 90g	●	29.7	n/a	120	1.5	0.3
Zucchini: *see* Courgettes						

TIP: Roast chunks of Mediterranean vegetables in a teaspoon of olive oil at 200°C/gas mark 6 for about 30 minutes, stirring a couple of times.

VEGETARIAN

The GL diet is perfect for vegetarians, and can easily be adapted to suit vegans as well. Watch the amount of bread you eat, pay attention to the quantity of nuts and monitor cheese levels, as some vegetarian cheeses are particularly high in fat. Use tofu or soya protein – tofu for preference, as it is low rather than medium GL. As with non-vegetarian ready meals, read the ingredients on vegetarian ones carefully, checking fat and sugar levels.

TIP: Make a delicious high-protein salad dressing by blending together some tofu, fresh herbs like coriander or basil, lemon juice and seasoning.

Food type	GL	Carb (g)	Fibre (g)	Cal (kcal)	Pro (g)	Fat (g)
Baked beans with vegetable sausages, 200g		24.4	5.8	210	12	7.2
Burgers:						
brown rice & tofu burgers, each		10.1	3.2	184	12.2	10.6
carrot, peanut & onion burgers, each		23.5	4.0	251	8.9	13.5
organic vegeburgers, each		27.7	2.3	238	3.1	12.7
savoury burgers, each		9.9	2.6	162	11.1	8.6
soya and black bean burgers, each		11.7	4.5	158	9.5	8.1
spicy bean burgers, each		30.9	7.6	234	7.3	9.9
vegetable burgers, each		20.8	1.7	179	2.3	9.6
Cauliflower cheese, 100g		22	–	365	18	23
Cheese, vegetarian:						
Double Gloucester, 25g		–	–	101	6.2	8.5
mild Cheddar, 25g		–	–	103	6.4	8.6
Red Leicester, 25g		–	–	100	8.1	8.4
Cornish pasty, each		37.3	2.0	452	11	28.9
Falafel, 4 (100g)		23.3	7.6	220	8	10.5

TIP: Marinate chunks of plain and smoked tofu, onion, peppers, tomatoes and button mushrooms in a teaspoon each of soy sauce (shoyu) and wine vinegar, plus a little Dijon mustard. Thread the tofu and vegetables on skewers, brush lightly with oil and barbecue or grill.

Food type	GL	Carb (g)	Fibre (g)	Cal (kcal)	Pro (g)	Fat (g)
Hummus, 2 tbsp	●	3.3	n/a	53	2.2	3.6
Lentils, 115g:						
green/brown, boiled	●	19.4	n/a	121	10.1	0.8
red, split, boiled	●	20.1	n/a	115	8.7	0.5
Macaroni cheese, individual	●	67	2.4	470	17	15
Nut roast, 100g:						
courgette & spiced tomato	●	12.5	4.9	208	11.7	12.3
leek, cheese & mushroom	●	13.2	4.1	240	13.2	14.9
Onions & garlic sauce, 100g	●	7.7	0.9	37	1.4	0.1
Pâté, 50g:						
chickpea & black olive	●	7.8	2.2	90	3.1	5.2
herb	●	3.0	–	83	3.5	8
herb & garlic	●	3.5	n/a	109	3.5	9
mushroom	●	3	n/a	107	3.5	9
red & green pepper	●	4.5	–	111	3	9
spinach, cheese & almond	●	3.2	1.2	86	3.6	6.6
Polenta, ready-made, 100g	●	15.7	n/a	72	1.6	0.3
Quorn, myco-protein, 100g	●	1.9	–	92	14.1	3.2
Ravioli in tomato sauce, (meatfree), 200g	●	26.4	0.6	146	6.2	1.6

TIP: Choose soya milk rather than rice milk, but avoid flavoured ones – they are all medium GL and high in calories. Sweetened soya milk, despite the low GL, is also significantly higher in calories than the unsweetened version.

Food type	GL	Carb (g)	Fibre (g)	Cal (kcal)	Pro (g)	Fat (g)
Red kidney beans:						
small can (200g)	●	27	12.8	182	16.2	1
boiled, 115g	●	20	n/a	118	9.7	0.6
Rice drink, 240ml:						
calcium enriched	●	23	–	120	0.2	2.9
vanilla	●	22.8	–	118	0.2	2.9
Roast vegetable & tomato pasta, 97% fat-free, each	●	56	–	300	10	3.7
'Sausage' rolls, 100g	●	28.2	2.5	273	9.7	13.5
'Sausages', 100g (2 sausages)	●	8.6	1.2	252	23.2	13.8
spicy Moroccan	●	12.7	4.0	147	9.1	8.4
tomato & basil	●	9.3	3.2	147	8.6	9.8
Soya bean curd: *see* Tofu						
Soya chunks:						
flavoured, 100g	○	35	4	345	50	1
unflavoured, 100g	○	35	4	345	50	1
Soya curd: *see* Tofu						
Soya flour:						
full fat, 100g	○	23.5	n/a	447	36.8	23.5
low fat, 100g	○	28.2	n/a	352	45.3	7.2
Soya milk:						
banana flavour, 240ml	○	25.2	2.9	180	8.6	5

TIP: Many vegetarian ready meals and processed foods are high in trans fats; watch out for hydrogenated fat in the list of ingredients.

Food type	GL	Carb (g)	Fibre (g)	Cal (kcal)	Pro (g)	Fat (g)
Soya milk, *contd*:						
chocolate flavour, 240ml	●	25.7	2.9	194	9.1	5.8
strawberry flavour, 240ml	●	18.5	2.9	154	8.6	5
sweetened, 240ml	●	6	Tr	103	7.4	5.8
unsweetened , 240ml	●	1.2	1.2	62	5.8	3.8
Soya mince:						
flavoured, 100g	●	35	4	345	50	1
unflavoured, 100g	●	35	4	345	50	1
Spaghetti 'bolognese', (meatfree) 200g	●	26.2	1.4	172	6.2	4.8
Sweet pepper sauce, 100g	●	4.3	0.5	89	1.5	7.2
Tofu (soya bean curd), 100g:						
smoked	●	1.0	0.3	148	16	8.9
steamed	●	0.7	n/a	73	81	4.2
steamed, fried	●	2	n/a	261	23.5	17.7
tangy, marinated	●	2.0	0.4	70	7.9	3.4
Vegetable biryani, each	●	74	–	690	12	38
Vegetable granulated stock, 30g	●	12	0.3	60	2.6	0.2
Vegetable gravy granules, 50g	●	29.7	1.6	155	4.2	2.1
Vegetable sauce, 100ml	●	7	2.5	59	2	2.6
Vegetable stock cubes, each	●	1.4	Tr	45	1.4	4.1

TIP: A dairy-free smoothie can be made by blending tofu with strawberries and a teaspoonful of honey. Whizz until smooth and drink immediately.

Food type	GL	Carb (g)	Fibre (g)	Cal (kcal)	Pro (g)	Fat (g)
Vegetable pasty, each	●	29.9	1.8	188	4.4	5.7
Yoghurt-tofu organic, 100ml:						
peach & mango	●	20.5	1.5	128	4.8	2.8
red cherry	●	20.1	1.5	125	4.8	2.8
strawberry	●	19.5	0.3	135	4.8	0.3-

TIP: Make an aubergine dip. Bake a whole, large, trimmed aubergine – prick it with a fork several times – at 180°C/gas mark 4 until soft. Peel it and chop the flesh; put this in a blender with 4 tablespoons low-fat natural yoghurt, a squeeze of lemon juice, 2 tablespoons of tahini, some parsley and a chopped clove of garlic. Blend until smooth, season if necessary and serve with raw vegetable sticks.

FAST FOOD

Most fast food is high GL, but you can make some compromises which will help your diet. Don't, for example, eat the hamburger bun; remove any batter from chicken or fish; avoid salad dressings; anything involving potatoes – no French fries, then – and all milkshakes and fizzy drinks. With sandwiches, be very careful in your choice of filling and check out any 'diet' options available, reading the ingredients carefully. Packaged salads are often already dressed and can contain high-calorie, high-GL ingredients like pasta or croûtons.

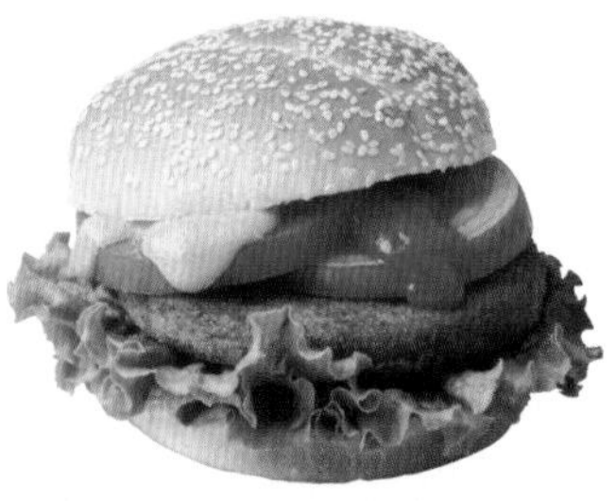

TIP: Never order anything, even drinks, super size. Watch the film *Super Size Me* and consider all the health problems Morgan Spurlock developed after just 30 days on a fast-food diet.

Food type	GL	Carb (g)	Fibre (g)	Cal (kcal)	Pro (g)	Fat (g)
Burgers/Hotdogs						
BBQ pork in a bun	●	67.9	3.6	555	30.2	19.4
Bacon & egg in a bun	●	32.3	1.7	345	18.8	15.49
Bacon in a bun	●	32.3	1.7	230	10.3	6.7
Bacon cheeseburger	●	32.3	1.7	345	19.1	15.3
Cheeseburger, each	●	33.1	2.5	315	16.7	13.1
Frankfurter:						
in a bun	●	33.5	2.2	410	21.8	22.4
in a bun with cheese	●	33.5	2.2	455	21.8	25.9
Half-pounder	●	42.3	6.7	840	51.2	51.5
Hamburger (85g)	●	32.8	2.5	253	13.1	7.7
Quarter-pounder	●	37.1	3.7	423	25.7	19
with cheese	●	37.5	3.7	516	31.2	26.7
Spicy beanburger	●	68.7	16.9	520	16.1	22
Veggie burger	●	46	7	420	23	16
Chicken						
Chicken chunks & chips	●	79.9	4.2	770	27.4	38
Chicken dunkers, portion	●	4.3	0.2	55	4.1	2.4
Chicken in a bun	●	42	1.9	435	16.3	22.2
Chicken nuggets (6)	○	7.9	1	208	14.2	13.3

TIP: Remember that a standard portion of French fries from many fast-food outlets can contain as many calories as an entire meal. And they are also very high in saturated and trans fats.

Food type	GL	Carb (g)	Fibre (g)	Cal (kcal)	Pro (g)	Fat (g)
Chicken strips, portion	●	3	0.2	64	4.8	3.7
Chicken wings, portion	●	3	2.3	466	40	32.7
Fish						
Cod, in batter, fried	●	11.7	n/a	247	16.1	15.4
Fish and chips	●	43.5	3.9	465	27.5	20.1
Fish in a bun	●	62.8	3.4	510	34.2	13.5
Plaice, in batter, fried	●	12	n/a	257	15.2	16.8
Rock salmon/dogfish, in batter, fried	●	10.3	n/a	295	14.7	21.9
Skate, in batter, fried	●	4.9	n/a	168	14.7	10.1
Pizza/Pasta						
Cannelloni, per portion	●	38.7	n/a	556	20.9	35.4
Deep-pan pizza, per slice:						
Margherita	●	31.5	n/a	256	13.5	8.5
Meat Feast	●	28	n/a	266	13	11.3
Supreme	●	29.6	n/a	257	13.1	9.6
Vegetarian	●	14.8	n/a	136	6.9	5.6
Lasagne, per portion	●	62.4	9.3	669	39.4	29.2
Medium-pan pizza, per slice:						
Ham & Mushroom	●	34	n/a	269	13	10.2

TIP: You can reduce the impact of sandwiches by discarding the top slice and eating them as Scandinavian-style open sandwiches instead.

Food type	GL	Carb (g)	Fibre (g)	Cal (kcal)	Pro (g)	Fat (g)
Medium-pan pizza, *contd*:						
Ham & Pineapple	●	28	1.3	241	12.1	8.9
Margherita	●	37.5	n/a	291	14.4	10.2
Meat Feast	●	27.8	n/a	324	16.6	16.2
Supreme	●	26.5	n/a	297	13.7	14.6
Vegetarian	●	26.2	1.8	225	10.5	8.8
Thin crust, per slice:						
Cheese & Tomato	●	18.2	1.7	126	6.7	2.9
Full House	●	18.9	1.3	183	9.3	7.8
Mixed Grill	●	19.6	1.7	177	9	6.9
Pepperoni	●	20.6	1.4	187	9	7.6
Tandoori Hot	●	18.7	1.9	138	8.2	3.5
Thin crust, per pizza:						
American	●	87.3	n/a	753	35.3	32.4
Fiorentina	●	88.4	n/a	740	38.22	27.5
Four Cheese	●	87.2	n/a	636	29.4	22.1
Ham & Mushroom	●	87.4	n/a	665	34.9	22.8
Mushroom	●	87.5	n/a	627	30.1	20.6
Tomato Bake, per portion	●	92.9	5.5	653	27.1	21.6
Tortellini, per portion	●	91.9	n/a	1116	26.9	71.3
Side Orders						
Fries, regular portion	●	28.3	2.8	206	2.9	9
Fries, large portion	●	33.3	2.4	550	36.2	30.3
Garlic bread, portion	●	55.4	n/a	407	10.1	16.1

Food type	GL	Carb (g)	Fibre (g)	Cal (kcal)	Pro (g)	Fat (g)
Garlic bread with cheese, portion	●	43.2	n/a	587	31.3	32.2
Garlic mushrooms, portion	○	31.6	n/a	240	5.5	10.1
Hash browns	○	15.8	1.7	138	1.4	7.7
Potato skins, portion	●	32	n/a	571	36.2	34.2
Salade Niçoise, per portion	●	65	n/a	729	40	37
Drinks						
Milkshake, vanilla, regular, each	●	62.7	–	383	10.8	10.1
Dips						
BBQ Dip, portion	●	9.4	n/a	39	0.4	0.1
Cheesy Bites:						
Cheddar	○	28.7	n/a	319	8.5	18.9
Tomato & Cheddar	○	26.9	n/a	308	8.2	18.6
Garlic & Herb Dip, portion	●	6.21	n/a	280	1.29	27.75
Ranch Dip, portion	●	3.8	n/a	489	3.2	51
Meals						
All-day breakfast	●	46	3.7	715	30.3	49.5
Egg & chips	●	32.5	2.7	490	20.8	30.6

TIP: If you are faced with pizza, have the smallest slice you can and fill up with salad. Avoid any salads with high GL ingredients as well as fat-laden dressings.

Food type	GL	Carb (g)	Fibre (g)	Cal (kcal)	Pro (g)	Fat (g)
Mixed grill	●	46.4	3.9	770	36.7	49.1
Spicy Chicken Bake, portion	●	80.7	–	499	18.5	12.4
Sandwiches and Wraps						
Cheese & pickle, per pack	●	51	3.8	341	16	8.1
Cheese & tomato, per pack	●	42	4.4	288	20	4.6
Chicken & ham, per pack	●	34	3.2	294	25	6.4
Chicken salad wrap, per pack	●	22	1.7	152	9.4	3.1
Egg mayonnaise & cress, per pack	●	47	3.7	323	23	4.8
Egg salad, per pack	●	44	2	304	13	8.4
Flatbread:						
chicken tikka	●	24	0.7	172	11	3.6
Peking duck	●	29	1.9	169	7.4	2.6
spicy Mexican	●	24	1.9	153	8	2.7
tuna	●	19	1.3	123	8.8	1.3
Ham & Double Gloucester, per pack	●	35	4.5	307	20	9.7
Ham, cheese & pickle, per pack	●	33	5	296	22	8.4
Ham & cream cheese bagel, per pack	●	45	2.4	319	19	7
Mini sushi selection, per pack	●	53	4.1	293	9.6	4.7
Prawn mayonnaise, per pack	●	42	5	287	19	4.6
Roast chicken, per pack	●	32	6.5	297	28	6.6
Roast chicken salad, per pack	●	40	8.8	317	26	5.9

Food type	GL	Carb (g)	Fibre (g)	Cal (kcal)	Pro (g)	Fat (g)
Salmon & cucumber, per pack	●	34	5.2	272	18	6.8
Toasted tea cake & butter	●	35.2	1.7	245	5.8	9.8
Tuna & cucumber, per pack	●	41	3.5	307	24	5.3
Tuna & sweetcorn, per pack	●	47	3.7	323	23	4
Tuna melt, per pack	●	33	2.6	258	21	4.7

TIP: Fish is good for you, but not if it's covered in batter. Take the batter off any fried fish if you can't avoid eating it altogether. Recent research suggests that using vinegar can help to reduce the impact on your digestion, so choose that rather than ketchup.

Putting it into Practice

LOW-GL MENU IDEAS

All the GL recipe books contain plenty of recipes and menu suggestions, but here are some other simple, hassle-free ideas. Adapt your favourite recipes for a GL diet by cutting down on the fat content, adding lots of low-GL vegetables and fruit, and boosting the fibre content.

Breakfasts

- Plain yoghurt, and one slice of wholemeal toast with yeast extract
- Porridge with a few dried apricots chopped and stirred in
- Kippers with lemon juice and black pepper
- Unsweetened muesli with natural, low-fat yoghurt instead of milk
- Egg-white or one-egg omelette with smoked salmon
- Chilled fruit smoothie made by blending low-fat natural yoghurt with frozen berries
- Reduced-sugar baked beans on one slice of wholemeal bread
- Poached egg on cooked spinach
- Grilled back bacon with tomatoes
- A slice of melon

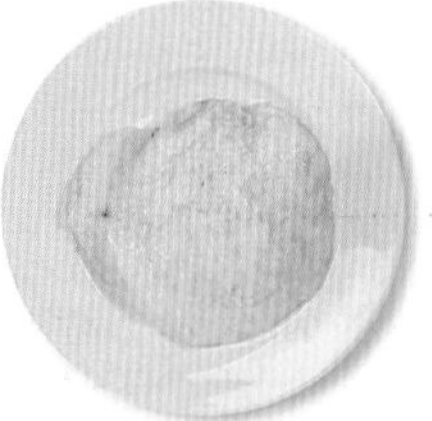

- Citrus fruit salad (no sugar but with a teaspoon of honey) with low-fat yoghurt
- Scrambled eggs with a slice of grilled back bacon
- Poached smoked haddock with a slice of rye bread

Lunches

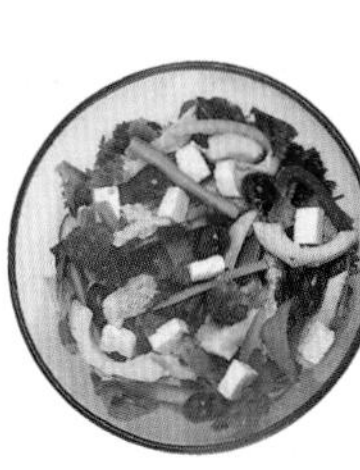

- Chicken soup (no noodles)
- Three-bean salad with tuna, lettuce and tomatoes
- Lentil and mushroom soup
- Smoked fish omelette with green salad
- Chickpea and courgette soup
- Greek salad – tomato, cucumber, onion, olives and feta cheese
- Open sandwich: smoked salmon, onion and pickles on rye bread
- Fresh tomato soup with torn basil leaves
- Tomato and avocado, sliced and sprinkled with finely chopped raw shallot and a few olives
- Lentil and onion salad, dressed and garnished with a hard-boiled egg
- Smoked mackerel salad, served with a slice of pumpernickel
- French onion soup, without the bread and cheese usually included but with a green salad on the side
- Tomato and courgette bake

Snacks

- Fresh fruit
- A small handful of unsalted nuts
- Homemade summer smoothie – blend natural low-fat yoghurt and strawberries together
- Crudités with a small helping of tzatziki (yoghurt, chopped cucumber and coriander)
- 16 olives
- Small bowl of cherries
- Low-fat yoghurt with fresh fruit
- Low-fat cottage cheese with raw vegetables
- Slice of watermelon
- A couple of dried apricots, chopped and mixed with 8 almonds
- Oatcake spread with hummus
- an apple and a small slice of low-fat cheese

Dinners

- Chilli con carne
- Grilled fish served with spinach and 2 or 3 baby new potatoes
- Steamed salmon served on a bed of lentils cooked with onions and herbs
- Roast vegetables and couscous with harissa (hot chilli sauce)
- Tandoori chicken or fish with crunchy green salad, onions and raita

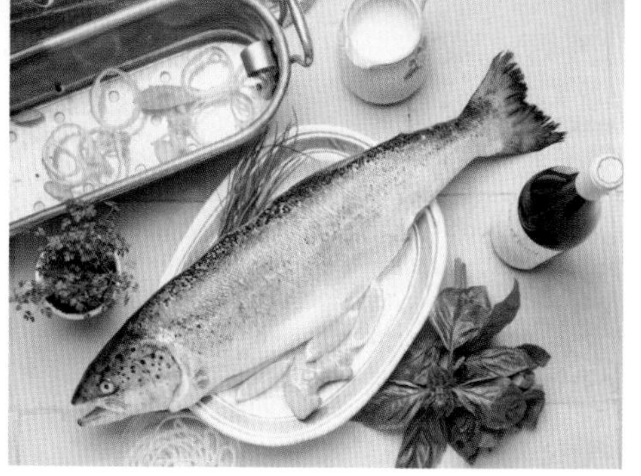

- Grilled salmon steaks with steamed broccoli
- Fresh tuna steak, grilled and served with a tomato, lettuce and onion salad
- Dhal with vegetable curry
- Trout with lemon, a few almonds and garlic
- Chicken, roasted with herbs and lemon
- Tofu and vegetable kebabs
- Grilled steak, trimmed of fat, with mustard and a large green salad

Desserts

- Baked apple filled with chopped, dried apricots
- Fruit fool made with low-fat fromage frais and sieved raspberries
- Strawberries with a tablespoon of vanilla ice cream
- Tropical fruit salad: papaya, mango, pineapple

- Selection of fresh fruit with nuts
- Baked egg custard
- No-fat Greek yoghurt with toasted almond pieces and a teaspoon of honey
- Stewed rhubarb, cooked with a little almond or vanilla essence
- Fruit salad of mixed berries served with raspberry purée
- Pears poached in wine and orange juice, dusted with cinnamon
- Slices of mixed melons: watermelon, galia, honeydew, cantaloupe
- Peach halves, warmed under the grill then scattered with toasted almonds

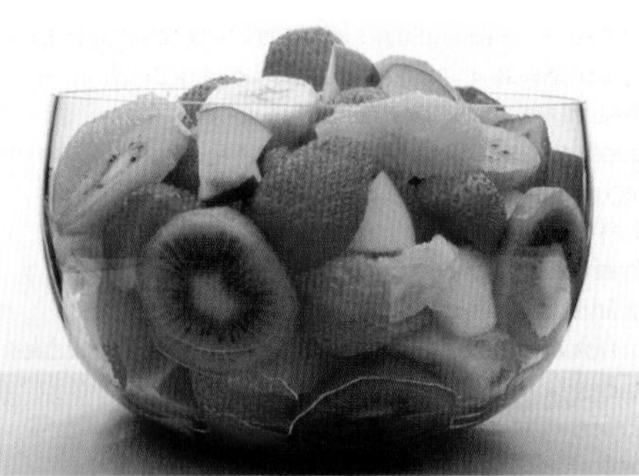

EATING OUT

Unlike most other diets, the GL diet can easily be applied to eating out once you understand the way it works and bear in mind its basic principles. Almost any kind of restaurant will have some dishes you can eat. You might need to do some substituting – have a salad instead of chips, extra vegetables instead of mashed potatoes – or ask questions about ingredients, but it should be fairly straightforward.

A few simple, general tips can help.

- If you know you are going to eat out, don't starve yourself during the day. Have a piece of fruit before leaving the house to take the edge off your appetite and make it easier for you to choose sensibly.
- For the same reason drink a glass of plain water at the restaurant before you place your order, maybe while you are looking at the menu.
- Keep choices straightforward; don't go for anything complicated or where you aren't reasonably sure what it contains. Ask questions if necessary.
- Watch the amount of alcohol you consume: resolve diminishes as alcohol intake increases.
- Try not to help yourself to fattening, high-GL nibbles from other people's choices (this can require extra willpower in restaurants where sharing is the norm, like Indian or Chinese places).

- Don't order everything at the beginning. Leave dessert until later; the chances are that you'll be full enough to do without.
- Eat slowly; if you've got too much don't worry about leaving some.

In this section, 11 well-known types of cuisine are listed alphabetically by their country of origin, along with advice about low-GL dishes you are likely to find on the menu, and foods you should avoid. There's information on fast-food restaurants on pages 202-8 and on packed meals on pages 230-4.

British

Bear in mind plate portion control – half vegetables, quarter other carbs and quarter protein – and choose relatively plain food which has been cooked simply. Avoid any fried food, asking for dishes that you know have been grilled; always trim the fat off meat and remove chicken skin.

Low GL – choose:

- Roast meat or poultry
- Porridge, oatcakes
- Dover sole
- Smoked haddock ('finnan haddie') with a poached egg on top

- Grilled fish, like trout or salmon
- Kippers
- Grilled steak
- Liver and bacon, if grilled

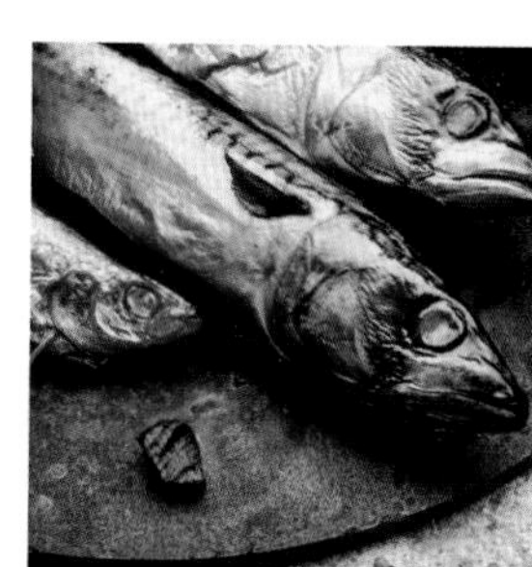

High GL – avoid:

- Bread
- Full English breakfast, especially toast or fried bread
- Fish in batter or breadcrumbs
- Potatoes, except for 2 or 3 baby new potatoes
- Pies, whether with a pastry or potato topping
- Yorkshire pudding and toad-in-the-hole
- Fatty sauces and those thickened with flour
- Rich puddings like sticky toffee pudding, steamed puddings or banoffee pie

Chinese

Chinese food is probably one of the most difficult cuisines for the GL dieter. The type of glutinous rice used has a particularly high GL, noodles are either medium or high GL and many of the sauces are sweetened or thickened. However, there are still some possibilities.

Low GL – choose:

- Clear soups, without wontons
- Peking duck, but no pancakes and go easy on the plum sauce
- Steamed, grilled or baked fish
- Prawns in their shells
- Plain spare ribs
- Tofu dishes
- Stir-fried vegetables and plainer dishes like beef with Chinese mushrooms or chicken with cashew nuts
- Soy sauce

High GL – avoid

- White rice, most kinds of noodles
- Prawn crackers
- Spring rolls, sesame prawn toasts, dim sum
- Sweet and sour anything
- Thick sauces
- The pancakes that come with Peking or crispy duck
- Lychees in syrup
- Toffee bananas or apples

French

There's been much discussion of the French paradox – why a nation that eats so much butter, cream, oil and bread should have a much lower rate of obesity than many others. However, this is beginning to change and the blame has been put on an increasing reliance on ready meals and convenience foods. In the past most French cooking was grounded in fresh fruit and vegetables bought at spectacular street markets; nowadays, particularly in the cities, eating pre-prepared food from supermarkets is much more common. In French restaurants generally, opt for the plainer dishes and decline the bread.

Low GL – choose:

- *Moules marinières* – mussels in a simple wine and onion sauce

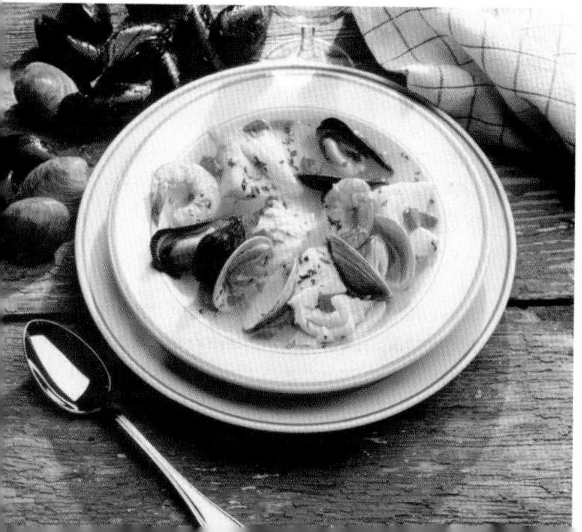

- French onion soup, but without the bread and cheese normally included
- Crudités – strips of raw vegetables
- Salads, such as Niçoise
- Grilled steak or fish
- *Cassoulet* – a haricot bean and meat stew, but not if it is topped with breadcrumbs
- Omelette and green salad
- *Bouillabaisse* – fish stew/soup, but decline the rouille sauce

High GL – avoid:

- Bread
- Cream sauces, creamy soups
- Potatoes and chips
- Patisserie and cakes
- Crêpes
- Pastry – savoury quiches, anything *en croûte* (in pastry), fruit tarts
- Rich desserts

Greek

Greek food is often perfect for the GL dieter. Many mezze, the 'little dishes' served as appetisers, are an excellent choice, and you can build a whole meal from them. There is normally plenty of grilled meat and fish as well as salads, and olive oil is generally used in cooking. Watch out for pitta bread and sticky puddings; 'Turkish' coffee often contains a lot of sugar, too.

Low GL – choose:

- *Horiatiki salata* – classic Greek salad with cucumber, onion, feta, olives and tomato
- Hummus with raw vegetables
- *Fasolia* – bean soup with vegetables
- *Gigantes plaki* – large butter beans cooked in a tomato sauce
- Grilled fish, seafood and meat
- Kebabs
- *Stifado* – beef casseroled with onions and tomatoes

High GL – avoid:

- Pitta bread
- *Dolmades* – stuffed vine leaves
- *Spanakopitta* – a spinach and feta pie made with filo pastry
- Anything deep-fried, like calamari (squid)
- *Kheftedes* – meat balls
- Moussaka
- Any spicy sausages; they are mostly high in fat
- Sweet puddings, especially baklava

Indian

Many Indian dishes are fine for GL dieters. The problem is that many are also very high in calories, so choose carefully and try to avoid anything with a very thick, creamy sauce. Rice, and all its variations, is another problem area, as are breads and the like, whether made of gram flour (chickpea flour) or not.

Low GL – choose:

- Tandoori dishes with salad and lemon
- Raitas – chopped vegetable, often cucumber, and yoghurt – and plain chutneys made from chopped vegetables
- Vegetable dishes as long as they're not potato based
- Dhals (made with lentils)
- Chana (made with chickpeas)
- Any baked meat or fish dishes
- Fresh fruit, not fruit canned in syrup

High GL – avoid:

- Deep-fried battered starters or those with pastry – bhajis, samosas, etc.
- Breads – naan, chapatti, poppadum, paratha, roti, puri
- Rice, including all biryanis
- Thick chutneys
- Potato dishes
- All Indian desserts and ice creams; tinned fruit

Italian

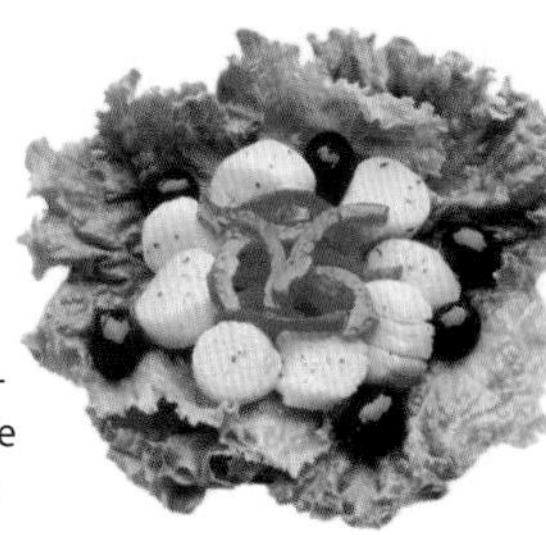

Italian food doesn't have to mean pizza or pasta, and there are normally several low-GL options. Even pizza or pasta restaurants will usually have some dishes to suit a GL dieter.

Low GL – choose:

- Varied antipasti – figs or melon with Parma ham; grilled vegetables, artichokes
- Thin soups, but not those containing pasta
- Salads, including *tricolore* – tomato, mozzarella and avocado – or seafood salads
- Grilled fish, poultry or meat
- Meat escalopes without any breadcrumb coating
- Fresh fruit

High GL – avoid:

- Breads, including garlic bread and bread sticks
- Pasta or gnocchi
- Pizza
- Risotto, which is usually made with a very high-GL rice, often arborio

- Polenta, made with maize flour
- Anything deep-fried, such as seafood
- Rich desserts

Japanese

Japanese food has a reputation for being healthy, and it is gradually becoming more familiar to Westerners. It is important to watch the rice, though, both as an accompaniment and as an ingredient in favourites like sushi. Flavourings are good: soy sauce and wasabi (strong horseradish) are both low-GL.

Low GL – choose:

- Tofu dishes, unless deep-fried
- *Teppanyaki* – grilled fish or meat with vegetables
- Sashimi – raw fresh fish with wasabi
- Steamed fish or poultry
- *Shabu-shabu* – thin slices of beef quickly cooked in stock, with vegetables
- Soya bean casserole

High GL – avoid:

- Rice and noodles
- Sushi

- *Tempura* – food (usually vegetables) fried in batter
- Anything in rice wrappers
- Anything coated in breadcrumbs and then fried
- Anything with mirin (sweetened sake) or miso (fermented soya beans)

Mexican

A lot of beans are used in Mexican cookery, but not all bean dishes are a good choice; some, especially refried beans, are very high in calories. Grilled meat or fish is often available, but don't be tempted by anything including rice, tacos or tortillas, or indeed anything made from maize flour – no nachos, for example.

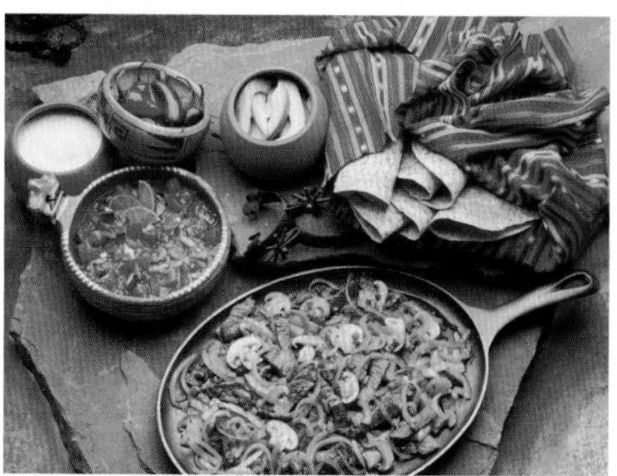

Low GL – choose:

- Guacamole with vegetable strips to dip in
- Tomato salsa
- Grilled fish, meat or poultry
- Black bean soup
- Ceviche – raw fish salad with avocado
- Chicken wings
- Chilli con carne – but hold the rice

High GL – avoid:

- Anything made with or involving tortillas
- Rice
- *Mole* sauces – thickened with chocolate
- Nachos
- Refried beans
- *Torta* – filled sandwiches and rolls
- Any pastries or desserts

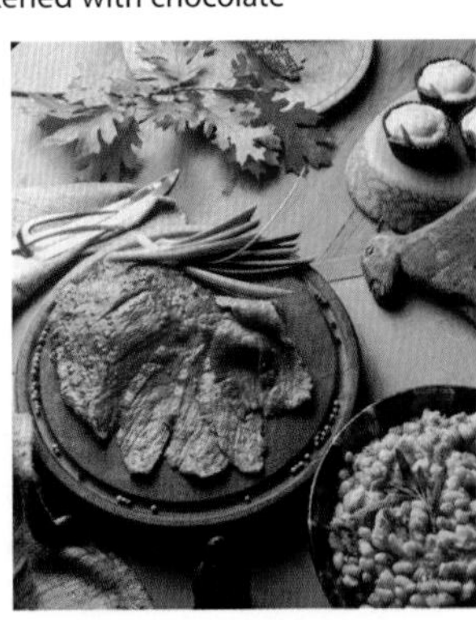

Middle Eastern

As with Greek food, you can easily make a whole meal out of mezze. Lentils, beans and nuts are widely used, salads are generally available and most Middle-Eastern restaurants have a good choice of grilled meats, poultry and fish. While a small amount of couscous is permissible on some GL diets, the quantity you are usually served in restaurants pushes it way off the scale. The same applies to tabbouleh, the bulgur-wheat and coriander salad.

Low GL – choose:

- Falafel – chickpea rissoles
- *Baba ghanoush* – aubergine dip with raw vegetables
- *Gibneh beyda* – white cheese (usually feta) dip
- Grilled meat or fish
- Kebabs
- *Ful midames* – a stew/soup made with dried broad beans and lentils
- *Kofta* – minced meat on skewers

High GL – avoid:

- Rice
- Bread
- Potato dishes
- Stuffed vegetables – because rice is usually included in the stuffing
- Pastries, both savoury and sweet
- Rich desserts
- *Lokhoum* – 'Turkish delight'

Spanish

Tapas – the traditional little appetisers of southern Spain – are now comparatively common and can offer some good low-GL choices, though you have to avoid dishes high in calories, like fried chorizo (spicy sausage). Portions are not always as small as they once were, either.

Low GL – choose:

- Olives and nuts
- White anchovies in vinegar
- Gazpacho – cold soup made with tomatoes and peppers – but say no to croûtons
- Grilled meats, fish and seafood
- Salads, such as *escalivada* – roasted vegetable salad
- Any omelettes except *tortilla española*, which has potatoes in it

High GL – avoid:

- Rice, including paella
- Anything deep-fried
- *Patatas bravas*, or anything which includes potatoes
- *Churros* – deep-fried strips of dough
- *Flan caramelo* – caramel custard
- Pastries
- Rich desserts
- *Turron* – nougat

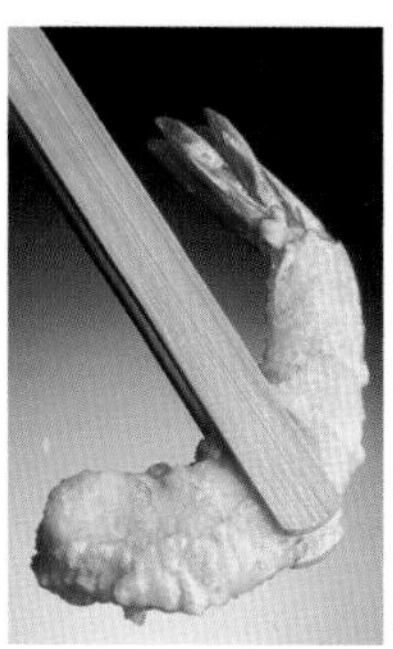

Thai

Stay away from the rice and noodles, and you should be able to have a low-GL meal at a Thai restaurant quite easily. Salads are generally available, and meat and chicken satay is popular, but be restrained with the peanut dip. Be wary of dishes cooked in coconut milk as they can be very high in calories.

Low GL – choose:

- *Tom yam* soups – clear soup with either chicken or fish and vegetables
- Salads, with vegetables, beef or fish
- Stir-fried meat and seafood
- Green and red curries, but without rice
- Steamed tofu dishes
- Chicken or meat satay
- Fresh fruits

High GL – avoid:

- Rice
- Noodles
- Any dishes that include rice (*khao*) or noodles (*sen*),

including *pho*, a popular soup

- Spring rolls
- Anything deep-fried

Packed meals

If you find yourself regularly eating away from home – and for most of us this means at work – then it's best to take a packed lunch. Sandwich bars, coffee shops and staff restaurants are all full of pitfalls that can blow your diet sky-high. Some suggestions for low-GL packed lunches follow.

Make sure you buy some decent packaging; no one wants a bag or briefcase full of lettuce leaves. Wide-mouthed flasks are ideal for soups; a drink flask can be awkward to empty and may retain a lingering coffee scent which would ruin a soup (and vice-versa). Try to carry salad dressing separately from the salad: though bean and lentil salads are best dressed in advance, this isn't true for leafy ones. A small plastic bottle is your best bet, so long as it doesn't leak.

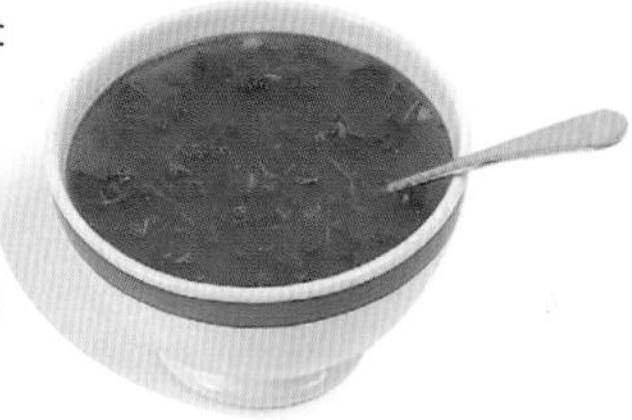

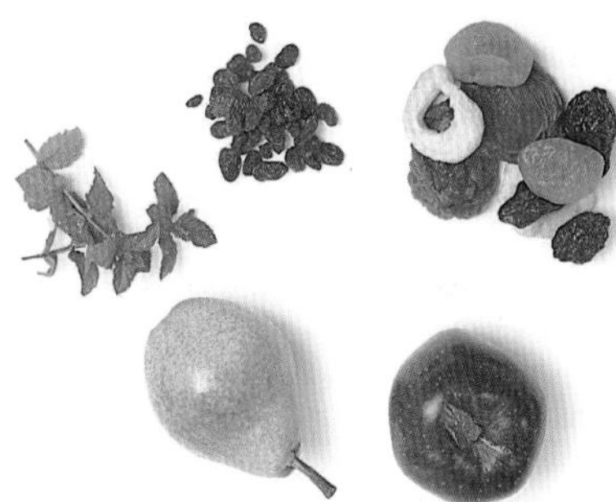

For many people a packed lunch means a sandwich. It doesn't have to, but if you are deeply attached to your sandwiches, then use thinly sliced rye bread or pumpernickel and restrict yourself to one a week. It may be worth taking the fillings separately; soggy sandwiches are very unappealing. Eating it as an open sandwich – take the top slice off and spread the filling over both – is an effective trick; somehow the meal seems larger.

Always take fruit. An apple is easily portable, and berries and softer fruits can be transported in a small plastic container. Emergency snacks can help you to stay away from the vending machines; take some olives, dried apricots, a few pistachios or a couple of oatcakes.

Avoid sugary carbonated drinks, boxes of fruit juice and flavoured mineral water (which often has a lot of added sugar). Go for plain water, tea, coffee – not in excess – herb tea or even hot yeast extract.

Fillings to put on your rye, pumpernickel or stoneground wholemeal bread:

- Hummus
- Smoked salmon and dill pickles
- Hard-boiled egg, chopped and mixed with low-fat mayo and a little chopped raw onion
- Slices of cold roast chicken with tomatoes

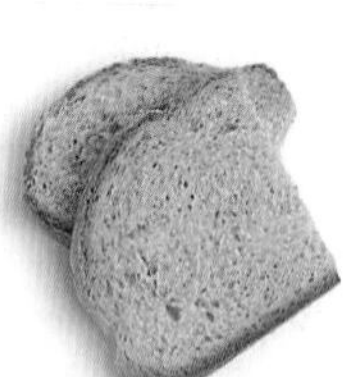

- Low-fat cottage cheese and lettuce leaves
- Low-fat cream cheese blended with tuna and a little paprika
- Cold lean ham, all visible fat removed, with mustard
- Lean roast beef with horseradish sauce
- Ripe avocado mashed with some vinaigrette
- Cold meat with homemade coleslaw – chopped cabbage, onion and carrot mixed with equal parts of low-fat mayo and low-fat natural yoghurt (carry this separately)
- Smoked mackerel pâté

Low-GL salads

- Chickpeas, spring onions, tomatoes, lots of chopped parsley, and an oil and lemon juice dressing
- Shredded cold chicken, beansprouts, spring onions and baby sweetcorn with a dressing made from a little soy sauce and lemon juice
- Strips of raw vegetables, plus radishes and cauliflower florets with a dip made from blended feta cheese and low-fat natural yoghurt
- Red kidney bean and walnut salad with chopped celery; add some rocket for an extra peppery taste
- Grated carrot with shredded cabbage and spring onions, dressed with a little olive oil and some squeezed orange juice

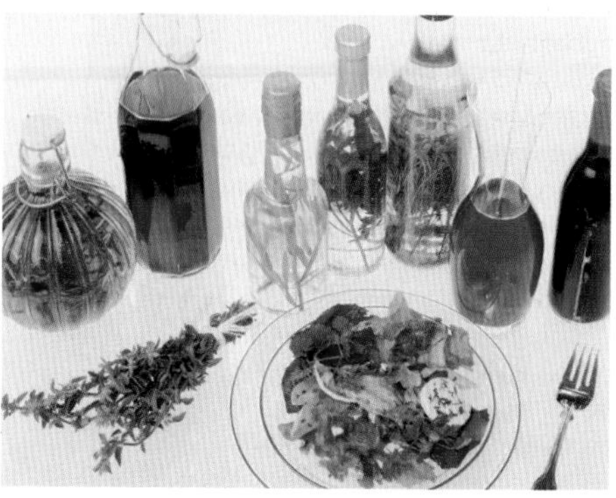

- Haricot beans and tuna with raw onions and black pepper; oil and balsamic vinegar dressing
- Multicoloured cabbage and pepper salad: shredded red and white cabbage, sliced yellow pepper, sliced onion, fresh green beans or a sliced green pepper with vinaigrette
- Lentil salad, with raw sliced mushrooms and onions; vinaigrette dressing
- Cannelini beans with finely sliced leeks, celery, red pepper and chopped tomatoes, with an oil and vinegar dressing including a little Dijon mustard

High-GL food and temptations to avoid:

- Any confectionery
- Crisps, no matter how small the packet
- Bags of salted nuts
- Biscuits and cakes
- Any fried food and shop-bought sandwiches. If you have no choice but to buy a prepared sandwich, go for the plainest one possible, on stoneground wholemeal or rye bread, and discard the top slice of bread
- Coffee shop cappuccinos and lattes – very high in calories

FURTHER READING

General Nutrition

Bodyfoods for Busy People, Jane Clarke, 2004
Collins Gem Calorie Counter, 2004
Collins Gem What Diet?, 2005
Collins Gem Healthy Eating, 1999
Collins Gem Carb Counter, 2004
Eat, Drink, and Be Healthy, Walter C Willet, MD, 2001
Eat Well, Live Well series, recipe books, various authors
Fat is a Feminist Issue, Susie Orbach, 1998
Food Pharmacy, Jean Carper, 2000
Healthy Eating for Diabetics, Antony Worrall Thompson & Azmina Govindji, 2003
A Good Life, Leo Hickman, 2005
Greek Doctor's Diet, Fedon Alexander Lindberg, 2005
Jane Clarke's Bodyfoods Cookbook: Recipes for Life, Jane Clarke, 2001
L is for Label: How to Read Between the Lines on Food Packaging, Amanda Ursell, 2004
Nutrition for Life, Ian W. Campbell, 2005
Patrick Holford's New Optimum Nutrition Bible, Patrick Holford, 2004
Think Well to be Well, Azmina Govindji, 2002
The Vegetarian Low-Carb Diet, Rose Elliott, 2005
Vitamins and Minerals Handbook, Amanda Ursell, 2001
You Are What You Eat Cookbook, Dr Gillian McKeith, 2005

The GI/GL Diet

The Holford Diet, Patrick Holford, 2005
The Holford Diet Low-GL Cookbook, Patrick Holford & Fiona Macdonald Joyce, 2005
The GL Diet, Nigel Denby, 2005
Eat Yourself Slim, Michel Montignac, 1999
Collins Gem GI Guide, 2005
Need to Know GI + GL Guide, Kate Santon, 2006
The GI Diet, Rick Gallop, 2004
The GI Diet – Shopping and Eating Out Pocket Guide, Rick Gallop, 2005
Living the GI Diet: To Maintain Healthy, Permanent Weight Loss, Rick Gallop, 2004
The GI Guide, Rick Gallop and Hamish Renton, 2005

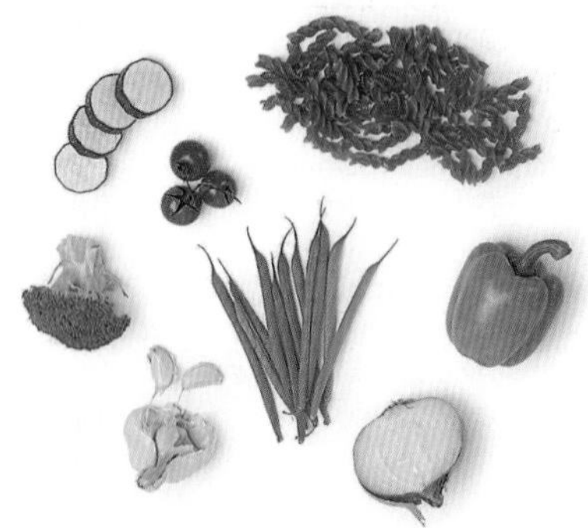

The Low GI Diet, Jennie Brand-Miller & Kaye Foster-Powell with Joanna McMillan-Price, 2004
The Complete Guide to GI Values, Jennie Brand-Miller, Kaye Foster-Powell & Dr Susanna Holt, 2004
The Low GI Life Plan, Jennie Brand-Miller & Kaye Foster-Powell, 2004
The Low GI Diet, Jennie Brand-Miller, 2005
The High-Energy Cookbook, Rachael Anne Hill, 2004
Easy GI Diet, Helen Foster, 2004
The GI Plan, Azmina Govindji & Nina Puddefoot, 2004
The G-Index Diet, Richard Podell & William Proctor, 1994
Antony Worrall Thompson's GI Diet, Antony Worrall Thompson, 2005
The Fat-Busting GI Angel, Gunter Schaule, 2003
The Simple 0–10 GI Diet, Azmina Govindji and Nina Puddefoot, 2005
The Healthy Low GI and Low Carb Diet, Charles Clark, Maureen Clark, 2005

USEFUL ADDRESSES

British Dietetic Association
5th Floor, Charles House
148/9 Great Charles St
Queensway
Birmingham B3 3HT
0121 200 8080

British Heart Foundation
14 Fitzhardinge Street
London W1H 6DH
0845 070 8070

British Nutrition Foundation
High Holborn House
52-54 High Holborn
London WC1V 6RQ
020 7404 6504

Coronary Prevention Group
2 Taviton Street
London WC1H 0BT
020 7927 2125

Diabetes UK
10 Parkway
London NW1 7AA
Careline 0845 1202960

Weight Concern
Brook House
2-6 Torrington Place
London WC1E 7HN
020 7679 6636

Women's Health Concern
PO Box 2126
Marlow
Bucks SL7 2PU
0845 1232319

USEFUL WEBSITES

www.dietfreedom.com (*Nigel Denby's site*)
www.patrickholford.com (*Patrick Holford's site*)
www.bodyfoods.com
www.weightlossresources.co.uk/diet/gi_diet (*wide range of information on boosting metabolism, burning calories and exercise)*
www.glycemicindex.com (*Jennie Brand-Miller's Australian website*)
www.gisymbol.com.au (*another Australian website*)
www.diabetes.org.uk/faq/gi (*Diabetes UK*)
www.waitrose.com/food_drink/nutrition/healthy eating/glycaemicindex.asp
www.gidiet.com (*Rick Gallop's website*)
www.ivillage.co.uk (*the Tesco website for diet queries*)
www.edietsuk.co.uk (*also used by Tesco*)
www.healthnet.org.uk (*Coronary Prevention Group*)
www.sainsburys.com/healthyeating
www.asda.com
www.bda.com (*British Dietetic Association*)
www.fdf.org.uk (*healthy lifestyle initiative combining healthy eating and fitness tips*)
www.weightconcern.com (*addresses physical and psychological needs of overweight people*)

PICTURE CREDITS

Photos © Getty Images:
Kevin Sanchez/Cole Group pp. 13, 52, 88, 106, 134
Chris Shorten/Cole Group pp. 14
Michael Lamotte/Cole Group pp. 18, 48, 78, 158, 223, 229
Ed Carey/Cole Group pp. 29, 31, 40, 70, 186
Dennis Gray/Cole Group pp. 39, 120, 128, 156, 214
Keith Ovregaard pp. 49, 74, 122, 150, 160, 178, 225
Allan Rosenburg/Cole Group pp. 64
Fred Lyons/Cole Group pp. 112, 196, 213, 233
Ernie Friedlander/Cole Group pp. 140
Jackson Vereen/Cole Group pp. 168, 217, 219
Patricia Brabant/Cole Group pp. 176, 202, 221, 224
Victor Budnik/Cole Group p. 227

Photos © Photodisc: pp. 9, 20, 22, 25, 46, 82, 96, 148

Photos by Christina Jansen, © Grapevine Publishing Services: pp. 10, 33, 35, 51, 54, 56, 58, 210, 211, 230, 231, 232, 236